The 7 Healing Chakras

The 7 Healing Chakras

Unlocking Your Body's Energy Centers

Brenda Davies, M.D.

Ulysses Press
Berkeley, California

Published by: Ulysses Press
P.O. Box 3440
Berkeley, CA 94703-3440
www.ulyssespress.com

Library of Congress Catalog Card Number: 99-64985

ISBN: 1-56975-168-4

First published as *The Rainbow Journey* in 1998 by Hodder & Stoughton, a division of Hodder Headline PLC

Printed in Canada by Transcontinental Printing

10 9 8 7 6

Editorial and production staff: Steven Zah Schwartz, Lily Chou, Jennifer Brontsema, Leslie Van Dyke
Indexer: Sayre Van Young
Cover Design: Leslie Henriques, Sarah Levin
Cover Photograph: "Dahlia" / SuperStock

Distributed in the United States by Publishers Group West and in Canada by Raincoast Books

The author has made every effort to trace copyright owners. Where she has failed, she offers her apologies and undertakes to make proper acknowledgment where possible in reprints.

This book has been written and published strictly for informational purposes, and in no way should it be used as a substitute for consultation with your medical doctor or health care professional. All facts in this book came from medical files, clinical journals, scientific publications, personal interviews, published trade books, self-published materials by experts, magazine articles, and the personal-practice experiences of the authorities quoted or sources cited. You should not consider educational material herein to be the practice of medicine or to replace consultation with a physician or other medical practitioner. The author and publisher are providing you with information in this work so that you can have the knowledge and can choose, at your own risk, to act on that knowledge. The author and publisher also urge all readers to be aware of their health status and to consult health professionals before beginning any health program, including changes in dietary habits.

*This book is lovingly dedicated to my mother and father,
my children, Keith and Lesda, and my love . . .*

Table of Contents

Acknowledgments

It's impossible to name all those to whom I feel gratitude. My parents, Hilda and Tom Todd, who gave me human life, loved me and shaped me in my formative years, set me on the course which led me to the point of writing *The Seven Healing Chakras*. Though my dad is no longer in his physical form, I thank them both from the bottom of my heart and give them my never-ending love. My children, Keith and Lesda, have borne with me through the hard times and I acknowledge with love and gratitude their pain, their patience, their love and their support. They have enriched my life in so many ways. I offer loving thanks to my best friend, Vickie, who has encouraged me, loved me and been the midwife at the birth of this book, plying me with tender sustenance and support. Her infectious humor has always enabled me to laugh at myself and keep a grounded perspective.

I thank Claire Gillman, my editor and now my friend, who sensitively taught me the skills of writing as she helped shape my verbose script into a readable text. Her skill has been inspiring. My thanks also to Rowena Webb for her tolerance and understanding. Scott Hunt has been my ever-supportive assistant, ready to do whatever he could to shoulder some of my clinical burden to give me space when I needed it. I thank Caroline Evans for tidying up my drawings and Rodney Paull for further refining them, Paulette Sharkey who was my long-suffering secretary at the beginning of the venture, and Melanie Marlowe who typed the script for me before I mastered my computer. Nigel Shakespeare who came in as my secretary quite late has nevertheless been ever eager to support my work. Thanks also to the team at Ulysses Press and to Briar Silich and Anna Cade at Hodder Stoughton. There are others too numerous to mention by name.

I thank all my teachers, and that includes everyone I have taught with whom I've had a simultaneous learning experience. I thank all those who have helped in my healing, and that includes all those I have had the privilege of guiding through their own healing. I thank all who have given to me, and that includes all who have allowed me to give. And for the great lessons which may have been wrapped in pain, and which I didn't want at the time, I give thanks. For often, those were the lessons that have moved me along my path the fastest and which were most essential to my growth. I give thanks for the unending love I have felt and for the generous care people have shown me. For the tolerance and indulgence I've received and the wonder of having so many amazing people accompanying me on my journey. There have been those who have accompanied me briefly and those who have been companions for much of this earthly life and before. There are those with whom relationships have changed and deep friendship remains. I have no doubt that we shall share other lifetimes in other guises.

To all those who have been the wind beneath my wings, I give my heartfelt love and thanks.

Brenda Davies
December 1999

Introduction: Birth of a Book

~

The Seven Healing Chakras is a child who has had a very long gestation—
it has been nearly born many times and then I've left it, preferring
instead to spend time with my patients. Finally, in late summer 1996,
I became physically unwell and this prompted me to listen to the messages I'd been avoiding for a long time. I took three months away
from my clinical work as a psychiatrist, and at last *The Seven Healing
Chakras* was born. As with my two biological children, its birth has
given me great joy and has made a big difference to my life. I wasn't
aware at the time that its birth might herald my partial retirement
from clinical work as I'd known it. Maybe on one level, I'd always
realized this would be the case and wasn't ready before. Perhaps that's
why I hesitated for so long.

The events that followed in my working life were unplanned and I
was unprepared for them. However, I strongly believe that God—or
the universe—always gets it right, and so it was, as usual, this time.

In the spring of 1996, after an exile of almost twenty years, I revisited
my beloved Zambia where I had lived and practiced medicine in the
1970s. As I was listening to the instructor giving his safety talk before
going canoeing on the Zambezi River, I realized that his words were
such a lesson for life:

"If you fall out of the boat," he said, "put your feet up, lie back and relax. Your life jacket knows which way is up. Let the river hold you. You won't drown." I'm sure God sent me that message affirming what I've always taught, knowing that I would need to remember it for myself soon enough.

The outcome of the various moves that took place after this trip was more than I would ever have thought to plan. I was reminded to do what I teach—that is, to live in the present, to send love and healing unconditionally wherever it needs to go and to give thanks for the opportunities created by the unexpected. The whole period showed me that I too need to listen to my inner voice on all levels—body, mind, emotions and spirit—to be true to my values and to refuse to live with compromise that prevents me from being who I am.

My desire to continue to work as I'd always done, and with the people, both staff and patients, whom I love and respect, had caused me to lose sight of my own growth and therefore of the opportunity to model a healthier way of being. Once back in focus, the rest became much more easy.

Holding on to what we think we want is not always the best thing. Accepting what the universe in its greater wisdom is offering us helps us to widen our horizons and moves us along our path with yet another lesson learned. Most bruising or pain is caused by attempting to cling on to what was—being unwilling to let go. We must allow the river of life to carry us along until we find where we need to be.

The Seven Healing Chakras has been my own journey, and though I was blessed with wonderful parents and good strong roots that have prevented me from being blown too far off course, I've also had my own agenda which I set long before this incarnation and upon which I'm still working. And when I've learned all I have to learn, taught all I have to teach, given all I have to give and received all I have to receive, my journey will be complete for this lifetime. I will be ready to leave my body and return to the place of freedom whence I came.

The journey may not always be easy, but it's exciting, and the further we go, the easier it becomes until we can eventually live on two levels at once, the human and the spiritual. As we clear the way, we encounter the most amazing gifts that we either didn't know were there, since they were buried under so much debris, or else we just didn't know how to use them. I assure you that the journey will lead you to a different place where you will learn to understand yourself and to be less judgmental of yourself and others. It's a place where joy becomes a permanent resident in your life and where access to whatever you call the highest possible force is as easy as it is wondrous. Whether you're actively working on yourself, or seemingly doing nothing, your growth continues. So why not decide to utilize every day fully? This Sanskrit hymn sums it up and may help get you on your way:

> *Look to this day for it is life; the very best of life.*
> *In its brief course lie all the realities and truth of existence—*
> > *The joy of growth,*
> > > *the splendor of action*
> > > > *the glory of power.*
> *For yesterday is but a memory,*
> *And tomorrow is only a vision,*
> *But today well lived makes every yesterday a memory*
> > > *of happiness,*
> *And every tomorrow a vision of hope.*
> *Look well therefore to this day.*

PART ONE

The Journey

ONE

Self-Discovery

～

Over the years, my practice of medicine has changed. I came to medicine comparatively late, having previously practiced as a pharmacist and been at home with my two children. Initially, I treated patients by dealing mainly with their bodies, then later, as a psychiatrist, I worked mainly with their minds. However, I'm also a spiritual healer.

I used to keep my spiritual healing practice entirely separate from my medical work, avoiding the derision of my peers and the disapproval of the medical profession in general. But, through personal experience, I've seen that spiritual healing is an essential and effective tool in the treatment of my patients, and over the last ten years I've come out of the closet, as it were. I have successfully combined all three disciplines. I believe that to achieve positive good health—and that's what I'm committed to doing—we must treat body, mind and spirit.

Healing the spirit offers both me and my patients an extra dimension. The body cannot be healed while there remains an unquiet mind, the mind cannot be well if there's emotional turmoil, and nothing can be whole unless the spirit is also considered. A holistic approach doesn't merely abolish symptoms—which are, after all, only an outer manifestation of inner pain—it allows for advancement across a broad front. Sometimes it takes longer to achieve tangible results this way, but the healing is more complete and the learning experience invaluable. At times, as patients live through their pain, it's a less comfortable process than it might be, for instance, using only medication. But, if the healing is done well, we should never have to go over the same ground again.

Spiritual health is our natural state and a goal achievable by each of us. Our task is simply to clear away the debris which obscures that reality at the moment. All we need is there within us. We're all wise and wonderful, and spiritual education, as with all education, is merely a process of rediscovering what we already know. It's often scary, however, to accept that nothing outside ourselves can make us whole and happy. We already are. True happiness, joy, peace and security are within us all. We just have to find them.

Having loving, like-minded people around us makes our way more fulfilling, but the strength, the grace, the power belong to you and you alone. To give away that power to anyone else, be it therapist, psychiatrist, lover, family or state, is to undermine our own spiritual worth. True loving is about empowering the beloved as we ourselves celebrate our own power. Beware of gurus who refuse to share their knowledge and therefore fail to empower the pupil.

The Seven Healing Chakras is a guide to spiritual health. It takes you on a journey through the chakras, the energy centers of the body. It shows how life events, pain and emotional disturbance set up blocks that prevent the free and natural flow of energy, leading to dis-ease— not only through our physical body, but also through our emotional and spiritual bodies, which jointly govern our total well-being. Each chakra is described and discussed in some detail before we look at the effects of disturbance in each area and at ways to let the energy flow.

New Perspectives

This book can only make sense to you if you're willing to let go of the restricted and rigid way of thinking that most of us were taught as children. It asks you to restructure old ideas and embrace a new perspective. We're taught that there must be a logical reason for all things. That there must be proof if we're to believe in something's existence. But, just think, there are rainbows. There have always been rainbows. They existed long before we understood them. We don't have to know how they're formed to believe that they're there. Nor do they have to be ever-present for us to know they're real.

When we're ready, we can prove how and why they exist. We can learn about light—how it can be split into all of the colors of the spectrum and how the rainbow is formed by a scattering of those light frequencies. Our new knowledge adds to our appreciation of the rainbow. But it doesn't mean the rainbow itself was any less valid previously because we didn't understand it fully. Rainbows didn't wait to exist until humans understood why. Some of the concepts in this book are like that.

What I would ask of you first is that you try to think more laterally, that you accept the possibility that there just may be more to life than you previously thought. We've generally been taught to focus and think in an orderly way, which is fine and essential to get us through life. What I'm suggesting, however, is that you learn to see more of the picture at any one time. At the moment, your eyes are focusing on the words on this page. You are looking out of your eyes at the print. But you're simultaneously aware of what there is in your peripheral field of vision. You can learn to see all of that field at once by softening your focus and simply allowing the whole field to enter your eye. It's almost as though the process were reversed, and rather than you looking out, you allow the field of vision to flow in. Other experiences can be similarly increased by softening the focus and being willing to allow them to flow into you.

Thinking laterally is like this. Allow other possibilities to enter your mind. Just relax and let thoughts, memories and concepts float in. What you will have is a vision of reality that is much greater than before. You may not be able to hold these new concepts for long at first. You may find that ideas come floating in, but before you can grasp them, they're gone. This may leave you feeling frustrated but also with a strange sense of excitement because you know that something different, something special happened. The trick is to try not to grasp or capture anything. What you saw or felt or momentarily understood will come again. It will float into your consciousness again with that same gentle excitement. When you're skilled enough at just allowing it to happen, it'll flow in, giving you a new understanding without any real effort at all. Eventually, new concepts will come as fully formed knowings that will enhance your life.

Recently, a friend gave me a very useful gift. It's a device to put on my car that warns deer to stay clear of an oncoming vehicle. It just looks like a little piece of metal. It appears to do nothing other than sit there attached to the grille of my car. But it emits a pitch of sound far beyond what you or I can hear and protects both me and the deer from possible collision and harm. It functions beyond my usual sphere of experience. I can't hear what it does, but I accept that it does something. Even if you can't see or hear what I am talking about right now, please try to trust. Just as the sound emitted by that device on my car can be tested and proven to be there, so can most of the things that I will be talking about.

Research has been carried out by Dr. Valerie Hunt in the USA in laboratories under strictest conditions over the last few years and there's now scientific proof of the existence of the body's aura and chakras, which you will be working with. But long before such proof was available, there were people talking about their personal experiences, sharing with the world what they could sense, see and hear. You might take a look at Barbara Brennan's excellent review of scientific investigation in her book *Hands of Light*, and at *The Chakras and the Human Energy Fields* by Shafica Karagulla and Dora van Gelder Kunz.

The things I'll be describing and discussing in this book are as normal to me as the existence of the rainbow. And there are many whose vision is much better than mine. I try not to envy them, since I know I'm on my journey and day by day I have a better understanding and better vision than I had before.

Illness or Imbalance?

What I'm sharing here is an amalgam of my work over a period of more than twenty years—work with patients in a formal way as a doctor and counseling psychiatrist, and also as a spiritual healer. Over the years, I've learned to understand illness in a different—some may say idiosyncratic—way which crosses the boundaries of traditional medicine and diagnosis. I see illness as a reflection of the comfort, or rather the discomfort, of our soul, so treatment must address the soul as much as the body.

Illness is about something being out of balance. On some level, all is not well. And the symptoms of the illness can teach us very specifically where and what the problem is if we learn some new rules and a new way of looking at what our bodies and minds are telling us.

Often by the time we're willing to take a real look at what's happening, there's already been considerable deterioration, and this may be so with you right now. We're sometimes so reluctant to come to grips with what's happening that by the time we do so, completely ridding ourselves of the results of the imbalance may not be possible. But, whatever the problem, you can always improve on some level if you start to take responsibility for the illness and therefore for its cure.

Symptoms are the signposts to keep us on the path we need to tread. If I put my hand in very hot water the pain receptors in my skin remind me that this isn't a healthy thing to do. Pain receptors are very useful, and without them I'd do myself serious harm. The pain receptors in my emotional self tell me the same thing. If I put myself in emotional danger, I'm sharply reminded by my emotional pain receptors that this isn't the way to go.

Although I learn very quickly on the physical level and don't put my hand back in the hot water, for some reason it takes me longer to learn from the emotional signals. The same is true on a spiritual level. I may have warnings for a long time that all is not well and that what I'm doing is not spiritually wise, but most of us initially fail to heed the warnings of the receptors there, too.

Unfortunately, it's likely that we'll miss the lesson until our mental, emotional or physical self takes up the message and gives it to us in a code that we readily understand and are unlikely to miss. Often, it is only when we become physically ill that we really stop to take note.

But we can learn to pick the signs up earlier and reduce the risk of illness if we set up time and space to listen. *The Seven Healing Chakras* will show you how. By using the exercises and techniques in this book, not only will you be clearing the past, you'll also be learning new ways to heal yourself and move on. Once we start to "hear" on a spiritual level and are willing to act upon the signals we receive, not only do we become more aware and more prepared for whatever is happening, we begin to move along more quickly, attracting the things we want into our lives, and letting go of what's obsolete.

I know that I'm not alone in my understanding and I have no doubt that before long there'll be universal acceptance of the major role the spirit plays in our total well-being. Many extremely talented physicians, surgeons, gynecologists and psychiatrists are already marrying the traditional with the ancient in the treatment of illness, allowing prayer to be a major part of their work and encouraging recognition of the spiritual aspects of their patients and the extra power this brings to the process of recovery. The ease, duration and completeness of recovery and healing are greatly promoted by this extra dimension.

In fact, there are now departments in universities studying the phenomenon of prayer. There are some well-designed trials studying and assessing the difference in recovery of patients who have a spiritual belief or who are prayed with and for before they undergo surgery and those who aren't. The results are more than encouraging. In some cases, they're astounding.

This book isn't really about prayer however, or perhaps not prayer as we generally know it. But if you can accept that living kindly and with integrity is a prayer, smiling at a child and wishing her well is a prayer, sexual expression within a loving relationship is a prayer, tenderly caressing your baby is a prayer, making a loving telephone call is a prayer, then this book may well encompass prayer making. Learning to send out some loving energy from your heart and allowing this to be transmuted into healing energy to help someone get well is also a living spiritual practice—a prayer.

So are you ready to open up to your own power of healing? To ensure that your life is lived to the fullest? To achieve your potential? To live peacefully with a sense of inner security that no external force can take away? What about learning to heal yourself? Are you ready to take an active role in being really well on all levels—in becoming the best that you can be?

This book is about you healing you, but it isn't about blocking off other avenues of help. It's also about giving and receiving, for only in keeping this dynamic open and flowing can the energy we all need for positive health be available to us. A very important part of healing is about receiving. One of the major causes of illness is our energy being so blocked that we are unable to receive. So this book is also about self-responsibility. About me taking care of me and accepting that it's my responsibility to do so. About me being independent but wise enough to allow others the joy of giving to me, so long as what they're offering is wholesome and good for me. It's also about having the courage to say no if you believe that what's being offered isn't right for you. It's about being big enough to accept that rainbows do exist even if you can't see them yet, and allowing others the space to see and believe what they wish, without judgement or the need to make them see it the way you do. In the end, you can believe exactly what you wish. That's your prerogative. But how about suspending judgement for a little while?

Something has drawn you to read this now and you may find that your whole world changes as you start to take charge of your life, as you learn to understand yourself better and see yourself and others with greater compassion. I have no doubt that what is right for you will happen.

Your Journey

You are already on the journey. This is it. But you can now choose to proceed in a planned and effective way or to continue to stumble along without a great deal of control. If you're willing to trust a little and give yourself a chance, you can do it differently. If you're willing to look at the usual ways you sabotage your progress, you can learn to be aware of these tactics and avoid them.

Your empowerment as you heal will lead you to moments of joy and clarity which at first may seem elusive, but which will eventually permeate all things. Some deep pain may continue to need work but that cannot detract from the growing sense of peace and freedom you'll feel, which you'll learn to tap into whenever you need or want to do so.

At times of crisis we may forget, be overwhelmed by hurt, and regress— but that too is part of the journey. We're not meant to be perfect. Our stumblings remind us why we're still here—we still have work to do. Flipping out into old pain or past behavior neither negates nor invalidates the work you've done. It simply pinpoints where there's more to do, where there's still unhealed pain and where attention needs to be focused now. It prompts us to give ourselves love, compassion, understanding, attention and time until balance is again restored.

The aim of the journey is to achieve and sustain that state of balance— with a sense of joy in being who we truly are on every level. As you proceed, you'll probably find that you want to be with others who are on a similar journey and this will enhance the experience for each of you.

As you go, be patient and gentle with yourself. Growth isn't an easy process at first. It's no mean task to change old habits and alter lifelong ways of thinking; to rid ourselves of negativity while still remaining realistic; to keep a healthy skepticism where appropriate while allowing for the possibility that things can change for the better. Our plan is to awaken, cleanse and vitalize our energy and to learn to allow it to flow freely, bathing us constantly as it heals and invigorates us and keeps us in a state of harmony and balance.

Your motives for wanting to take this journey are also important and need to be examined before you begin. This journey of self-discovery will generate enormous power. But that power is to be used for your own higher good and with a sense of love and service to others. Without such a commitment to the higher good, there'll be only disappointment. Perhaps you could spend a little time reflecting on why you want to come along and then we'll begin.

My Own Journey

I've often joked that if ever I write my autobiography, I'll entitle it "The Rat-catcher's Daughter," for that's who I am.

My own journey in this lifetime began in a tiny village in the northeast of England as the younger of two daughters. My mother was a nurse, though she never practiced after we were born. My father would have loved to have gone to a university, but as one of fourteen children, it was impossible. Instead he became a highly skilled and much sought-after steel erector, working on high chimneys and church steeples. My parents married in the pre-war years with high hopes for the future. However, before the age of thirty, my father was cut down in his prime by severe head injuries during World War II. On returning home with temporal lobe epilepsy, he couldn't return to his previous job and instead spent the rest of his working life as the local rodent officer. There was little he couldn't do, however, and his need for independence drove him on to overcome many of his difficulties. He offered us a model of courage, dignity and North Country wisdom that continues to be an inspiration to me.

My mother was, and remains, a very loving woman and I remember sweet, happy days laced with laughter and affection as well as respect for her as our mother. She was very proud of us as we grew, and there was never any doubt that she held us in high esteem, which gave each of us self-confidence as we made our way in the world. Dad was less affectionate, rarely touching or kissing us, though he had his way of showing his great love for us. Only as I got older, well into my forties, did he become openly affectionate with me, though even then he would rarely say he loved me. One of my most precious moments with him was shortly before he died when in response to my usual statement of love for him, he replied, "Of course you do. We'll love each other till the end of time. Isn't that how it's supposed to be?"

Between them, my parents gave my sister and me the best upbringing they possibly could, with firm, strong roots, good values, a sense of pride in who we are and a philosophy of self-sufficiency and independence.

When I was a little girl—say four or five—I began to experience an interesting phenomenon which is difficult to describe. I felt as though I had love all around me, running through me and radiating from me. I would have to ground it in some way, usually by touching something or someone, like one of my animals or my mom. A strong, palpable current had begun to flow through me and, long before I knew anything about chakras, I could sense places in and around me where the energy seemed to halt briefly and then pass on.

And so my spirituality was born. I could feel so wonderful and full of love. I could use it with my animals, and did so regularly. Looking back, that's where the healing began, though neither I nor anybody else recognized it as such then.

It was years later when I was married with two children and had returned to the university to study medicine that a gynecologist I was working with pointed out that there was something different in the way I was with patients. The women I sat with and touched would need little sedation or analgesia. Even then, however, I didn't really recognize that healing had become a major part of how I practiced.

While living in Zambia in my thirties, I was fascinated by the power of the traditional healers who often had answers that modern medicine did not. I remember one patient who'd been in a traffic accident and had broken his back. We sent him home in a wheelchair with no hope of ever walking again. A few weeks later, he walked into the ward pushing his chair. He thanked us for doing what we could, but said that the village doctor had gotten rid of the bad spell and he was fine now! There are many similar stories that taught me lessons I've never forgotten and opened my eyes again to the power of healing.

The transition from physical medicine and surgery to psychiatry was a perfect part of the journey—from the body to the mind and back full circle to the spirit as I worked through my own process, clearing my own path. My two children were grown, and in 1984, having out-grown each other, my husband and I agreed that our long marriage should come to an amicable end. So I was free to become who I am.

At last I had the courage to stand up regardless of the derision of my peers and "come out" as a spiritual healer. I began to marry my excel-lent traditional training as a doctor with the ancient creative skills of the shaman. My practice responded with a phenomenal rate of growth. I had made a pledge to God long since, when I desperately wanted to become a doctor, that I would see everyone He sent to me, and this I did regardless of whether it appeared that I had the time or the energy. He always somehow gave me both.

It was only in 1996 that I at last acknowledged things had to change. At that time, I was a very busy psychiatrist running a hectic private practice in London, serving as Director of Clinical Development in a beautiful clinic in the suburbs, and running spiritual workshops and teaching internationally as time allowed. In my psychiatric practice, I was balanced between two worlds. On the one hand there was tradi-tional allopathic psychiatry, and on the other, healing and comple-mentary medicine. My own spiritual growth was also ever beckoning.

I'd been using healing in my practice for some years, my patients enjoying this extra dimension and the feeling of self-realization and control it would give them. For me, it allowed me to be who I am and left me energized and fulfilled. However, in the clinic I tried to use only modern medicine, feeling uncomfortable if I used alternative methods, which I knew were effective but which were incongruous with the philosophy of the hospital.

The place I could move to the bounds of spiritual healing was in my workshops, which I'd been running for nearly fifteen years. There I could work with spiritual energy and use ancient healing techniques and the power of love. I could see people respond in a different way as they became more whole, quickly and without the use of medication, mobilizing their feelings, healing old wounds, releasing energy and moving forward. The amount of love generated in those workshops was a privilege to behold. Unfortunately, I didn't have the facilities at the hospital to continue the spiritual work for the many who wanted to do so.

For a long time I struggled with my heart and my conscience, trying to find the way forward that would accommodate my needs, the needs of the patients and of the clinic. These were the spiritual messages I failed to heed, and since I also sidestepped the emotional pain I felt in being unable to practice as I knew I should, the pain finally filtered down to the physical level. I became ill and the message could no longer be ignored.

Finally, forced to take time off for the first time in over twenty years, I was able to stand back and see the cause of my distress. I was doing to myself what I'd seen many of my patients do over the years. I was trying to do what was best for everyone. Trying to be there for my patients and for the clinic and the staff, for whom I have great regard, and, in the end, neglecting what was right for me.

I finally accepted that I had to make a move toward using my spirituality every day. To make it not only my way of being in my personal life, but also my way of working, even if that meant severing the ties with the wonderful people I worked with. I could no longer compromise myself by restricting my own potential in a bid to help others achieve theirs. Basically, I had to help myself before I could truly help others. Leaving the clinic meant an enormous shift financially and emotionally, but it also meant getting back in line with my integrity, allowing me to be myself and reclaiming a clinical freedom that I'd allowed to erode over the years.

I recount this because many of the people who knew me and worked with me then were astounded by the events of that time: first that I was ill, which seemed to call into question the healing I teach; then, that I took three months away to rest and think; and then that such a major move occurred. More than that, however. Some of my patients had always felt I had my life all worked out and was able to live constantly in the way that I would teach. It is, I hope, refreshing to see that an unhealthy way of being can creep up on anybody, almost without notice, and that sometimes the only way to see it is to stand back and evaluate the situation.

While recovering in South Carolina in the midst of this change and still feeling the pain, I met a clinical psychologist, Dr. Helen Barry. In her late seventies and looking not a day over sixty-five, she shared with me much of her wisdom. On one occasion she recounted how she had been having some art lessons and her teacher had suggested that she stand back to get a better view of her work. "Just get your nose out of the paint."

Those words have been very useful and I hear them in my mind often. Standing back from my life, as I was forced to do while I was unwell, was just what I needed to give me a better view.

I've always taught that messages come to us on a spiritual level first, where we may perceive them as a nagging discomfort. We know that something just isn't right. Often we're aware that we aren't living according to our own internal standards or values, that we're allowing ourselves to be compromised or aren't having the courage to stand up for what we know is right.

I heard the messages probably as early as 1993, but I still continued to work traditionally as I tried to make as few waves as possible for myself and my colleagues. To avoid consternation at work, I even avoided talking about healing and moved my workshops away so that I could still spend a week now and then working as I wished to. None of these moves was radical enough. I needed to trust the universe that I'd be fine, as over the years I've supported many others in doing. I also needed to trust that others would be fine. I needed to let go of the co-dependent attitude that made me worry about how everyone else would cope with my leaving.

This book is the result of my change of direction. It brings together what I've been teaching for most of my professional life and it comes equally from Brenda the psychiatrist, Brenda the spiritual healer and Brenda the woman. Brenda is happier now than she allowed herself to be for the two or three years preceding the change. The learning that took place during this time has also, I hope, enriched the book. One of my favorite sayings is that the universe always gets it right and so it is with the process I've just described. Obviously I wasn't ready in 1993, nor in the couple of years after, to make the leap I eventually made. It had to wait until all was ready and then the transition was easy. All the obstacles that had previously been in the way just rolled back, leaving the path clear and, with apparent lack of effort, I simply walked out onto it.

Some might say we could put our lives on hold forever waiting for the right time. I can't say that I agree totally. We can procrastinate, reacting to events while never seeming to initiate real change for ourselves. Or we can get into the driver's seat of our lives and move forward, pushing ahead to our intended goal. But we must be allowed to choose the time. Often, well-meaning friends, relatives, partners, therapists, psychiatrists and others seem to think they could live our lives better than we can! But we learn exactly what we need to and there's probably no better way than the set of circumstances we find ourselves in right now. The lesson of today is important and essential wherever we are. Nothing is lost. Nothing.

Making Changes

The fact that you're reading this book shows that you want to make some change and even if today's step is only to read this and do no more, that's fine. When you're ready, the rest will follow.

In wondering which way to go, what changes to make, just spend a moment now and then tuning in to what's going on in your body and in your emotional self. Do you feel drained? Are there some people you dread seeing because you feel low, lethargic or even ill afterward? Does spending time in some place or with somebody give you a headache? Do you sometimes feel anxious and afraid for no apparent reason? Do you feel lost and without direction? Do you feel as though you don't belong anywhere—and perhaps never have? Do you stay in abusive situations so long that, in effect, you become your own abuser? Do you have an illness that you would like to understand better and help relieve? If the answer to most of those questions is "yes," then you'd be wise to think of making changes.

Or do you have a light feeling? Are there people around you with whom you feel energized? Are there places or activities that leave you feeling elated and expanded? Do you have moments of feeling safe and comfortable? Is your body feeling good? Then these are also giving you a powerful message about where you need to be, with whom and doing what.

When you decide to make changes, it would be good to do so without guilt, with love to all concerned and with the affirmation that whatever you do is not only for your own good, but ultimately for the good of all. In that way, your move will be light and easy and you'll have the knowledge that you're acting from your highest and purest intention.

Sometimes there will still be a nagging feeling somewhere, usually in the region of your solar plexus. Sometimes we're still a bit out of focus with our plans and our integrity is being threatened a little (see Chapter 8, page 121. If that's so, stop and imagine you are looking through the lens of a camera. What needs to be gently adjusted to bring the picture back into focus again, to bring clarity? Take your time and you'll see where you need to proceed more slowly, or where perhaps you need to make a more radical adjustment. But do try to be clear that this isn't guilt or your need to be taking care of everyone else's feelings instead of your own. When you feel comfortable again, proceed. No one is timing you. No one is saying you have to make changes, do exercises or meditations anymore quickly than you feel capable of—or even at all.

We'll follow the natural progression through the seven main energy centers—the major chakras—from base to crown, and by means of both inspirational meditation and practical exercises, you may be led to a place of improved health and vitality. Though of course no claim is made to cure established illness, this book can aid in the prevention of disease and can promote self-healing. In all cases, if the steps are followed diligently, there should be an increase in self-confidence, self-esteem and well-being.

There is an emphasis on personal responsibility and the establishment of a new way of life incorporating spiritual (not necessarily religious) practice into your daily routine. For many years, most of us have abdicated responsibility for our own health and have been eager to leave it in the hands of doctors and others. This book is about reclaiming your power to heal yourself and make yourself whole.

The journey to wholeness should be fun even though at times it will not be free of pain. If there is pain, try not to resist. Pain is increased by resistance. If you slide into it, lean into it, breathe into it, it will be transient and will yield much in terms of growth. Allow yourself as much love and compassion as you can muster right now—both will increase, not only for yourself but for the whole of humanity as you proceed.

Come . . . become the best that you can be.

Enjoy!

TWO

Before You Embark

∾

The Seven Healing Chakras is a complete guide to self-healing. It is intended to help you take control of your health while remaining in partnership with your doctors or other medical professionals and complementary therapists. It is intended to help you learn more about your whole self—not only your physical self, nor indeed the emotional, intellectual, or spiritual self alone, but all of you.

If any one of these areas is blocked or unhealthy, achieving balance in the others is difficult. Sometimes we appear to have a problem in one department when really the issue is elsewhere. It may be, for instance, that you're complaining of a backache, yet you need to look at what you're carrying, psychologically speaking, and see how you can put that burden down. It may be that you're tearful and sad, feeling depressed when really you need to mobilize some anger or look in a more holistic way at your life. Being spiritually deficient can give rise to feelings of isolation and abandonment that need to be healed from the inside so you'll never feel isolated and alone again.

Many of us are stuck with a limited view of our totality, seeing ourselves as physical beings with a mind and feelings but nothing else. For some, even feelings hardly exist and the concept of us being spiritual entities is a foreign and ridiculous notion. This isn't a factor of intelligence or education. It may be that you're a young soul with much still to learn of the physical and material world, and therefore unable as yet to encompass the whole. It may be that hurt has prompted you to close down and become cynical, leaving you with a kind of tunnel vision in which a holistic view is impossible. Whatever your situation, by reading this book you're already on your path to your own higher wisdom.

As you progress through *The Seven Healing Chakras*, you'll learn to take care of your whole self, to clear blocks that have occurred as a result of the experiences you've accumulated in all your lifetimes thus far. It'll teach you new ways of recognizing and releasing energy so you can use it to your best advantage and be truly well. By "well," I don't just mean free of illness, but being positively well, having energy to spare and stamina that will last you all day and into the night if necessary. You'll find joy in the simple things that each day offers to every one of us, but that we often miss with our senses dulled and our eyes downcast on the only path we see before us. Life has so much more to offer than this.

You can learn to embrace your life and truly live it, guiding it to where you want it to go while all the time taking note of the spiritual, emotional, physical and mental signposts that are all along the way.

There's no reason we shouldn't be a great deal healthier than we are. Some illnesses may be completely reversed by self-healing. All can be improved to some extent, as can your whole life. Healing is not only about getting rid of disease when it already exists. It's also about preventing illness and promoting positive good health. But one of the main goals is to help us become the best we can be, finding our true path and fulfilling our potential. Having an early warning system that all is not quite right—and listening to it—is also useful. But so often we ignore the signposts. Just look at what I allowed to happen to myself in 1996. Even knowing and understanding doesn't prevent us from coming unstuck at times.

Being active, being vigilant and learning a new way of living that allows us to grow and live with joy is what this book is about.

Using This Book

The book is divided into ten chapters. Chapter 3 explains the principles of healing, auras, and the seven major chakras. Each of the remaining chapters is devoted to a specific chakra and includes exercises and meditations focusing on problems associated with these centers. Appendix A (mainly for therapists, but do read it if you feel you'd like to) explains how the major glands and nerve plexuses are related to the chakras, and Appendix B looks at evidence of etheric bodies.

You may decide to read the book once and then go back and work through it a stage at a time. You may feel that you can absorb one chapter very quickly and then need a long time with another. That's all right! Do it in whatever way you are comfortable. But . . . you *need* to do it all. Even if you find that your major block is at the first chakra, there will be some distortion further up the system, however minimal. Similarly, a block at the throat chakra will have affected all the others to some degree. You may find that because one area is blocked, you've been over-compensating in another. We're moving toward balance, so everything will need adjusting, even if just a little.

There's a self-assessment questionnaire at the end of this section (page 28) that will give you some idea of where your main blocks are located. However, try not to be too discouraged if you find there are problems at every chakra, nor too elated if you find that most seem clear— everyone, no matter how spiritually evolved, can benefit from a little fine-tuning.

Again, don't be alarmed or discouraged if you clear up one area only to turn around and find that it's blocked again. That's not surprising either. If you've been living a long time with a paucity of energy flowing through, you may find it difficult to live with absolute clarity for a while. A strong flow of clear sparkling energy is a very rich diet to cope with. Healing will only occur to the point at which you can deal with it. Miracles do happen but not everyone is ready for one. After all, your current situation and state of health and well-being are what you're used to, even if you don't like them very much. Also, you're still learning something from being there. Changes may have to be gradual. Sometimes it's very scary to let go of what you know and leap into the void. Be gentle and compassionate with yourself.

Whether you're just starting on your journey or whether you're well on your way; whether you're a professional using healing techniques in your work or you're just looking for a better way to live your life, *The Seven Healing Chakras* will offer you suggestions, guidelines and opportunities for growth. Some of the terminology may seem foreign to you. I hope it will all be explained as we go along, but if you're unsure of a meaning, there is a glossary on page 228 which will help you.

Nothing here is meant to replace any other help you're receiving. It's not intended, for instance, that you should stop therapy, or medication, or let this work interfere with anything else in your life unless or until you want it to do so. But as you work through *The Seven Healing Chakras*, if you do get that light excited feeling, then perhaps you could follow it and see where it takes you. For that is your spirit responding to your approach and welcoming your awakening.

Life can be full of the most amazingly wonderful things. It can be filled with love and laughter. It can be joyful, exciting and fill your heart with peace and pleasure. Even if thus far you've had a raw deal, it can get better, but you have to do the work. And if you aren't there yet, please don't think that I'm judging you and saying you haven't worked hard enough. I am full of admiration at the courage I see every day as people work on their issues. My heart goes out to them and sometimes I wish I could do it for them, but that's not my job. We have to do it ourselves. I never cease to be in awe of the strength some people exhibit. Often those with the worst histories seem to have the stamina to carry on working long after many would have given up. I tell them and myself that they had to learn coping skills the like of which I may never have because they had to survive.

And if you feel you can't go on one step further, take some time out and be gentle with yourself. You'll be amazed at the reserves you can draw upon. We can always go that bit further if we have to.

When you feel better you'll see that health and happiness are not dependent upon anything material, or upon anyone being in your life—though to have a compatible life-traveling companion is wonderful and there's a lot to be said for being prosperous. It's all about your inner self. About your own work, about your own growth. It's all about the magnificent being that you are and have always been. Sometimes depression, maladaptive behavior or illness is like a cloak we've become used to wearing—but we can take it off, and there underneath is the real thing.

What You Will Need

Let's look at the things you'll need to gather together before you begin.

Notebooks

It's a good idea to have a couple of exercise books. One is for you to write down affirmations (see Glossary) which you'll be creating as you go along; the other is to use as a journal.

Often writing for twenty minutes or so allows you to get to the nitty-gritty of what you really feel. It can be very revealing. But also, as you begin to deal with the past, a good way of clearing up the feelings is to write letters that you aren't going to send which allow you to have your say, to externalize what you feel; and this can be very therapeutic. These letters can go in the second book, so that you have a record of your journey.

There'll be amazing happenings—coincidences, you may call them—which are worth recording so that you can map your progress and eventually blow away any skepticism you may have begun with.

Angel Cards

Another thing you might like to try using is a pack of angel cards. These are a collection of tiny cards, each bearing the name of some quality or gift you might need at that moment, for example peace, trust, sincerity. The idea is to highlight it in your being and ask the appropriate angel to be with you to help you. When I mention angel cards at workshops, people usually titter: they think they've come to the wrong place and that this psychiatrist really is crazy after all. However, the same people a short while later will be the ones giving the loudest gasps when again and again they find that exactly what they need is reflected in this little oracle.

For those of you who have used the I Ching, an ancient oracle devised by Taoists in China, it may not seem so strange. An oracle allows us to ask questions or tap into the powers that are there at any particular moment in time to gain wisdom. Carl Jung used the I Ching regularly to aid diagnosis and, although I don't use it for that purpose, I've often used it in my own life to help clarify something I may have been struggling with. The angel cards can be used similarly although the process is much more simple. If with an open and pure heart and good intention you ask for what you need, you'll be surprised at the accuracy of the reply.

Angel cards can be purchased in most New Age bookshops or perhaps from shops that sell crystals and gemstones.

Tape Recorder

You'll either need to record the meditations or have a friend read them to you.

Sacred Space

A quiet place in which to work would be good. We'll be looking at making a safe place within yourself but, if possible, have a place to work that you can call your own, where you won't be disturbed and where you can put some objects that are significant to you and which help you feel at peace. Maybe some candles (be careful when they are lit and don't leave them unattended), a crystal or two, your books, a nice pen, perhaps some flowers, a vaporizer with your favorite oils (some are more appropriate to various chakras—we'll deal with that as we go), a photograph perhaps—whatever you'd like. If you don't have a room you can use, a little corner, or an armchair with a small side table will do. Even a box with a cloth over it can give you a feeling of a sacred space that's yours.

Crystals

Having the right crystals doesn't have to be a big deal or an expensive exercise. You don't even have to have any at all. If you want to, you can do all you need with a clear quartz, a small piece of amethyst and a piece of rose quartz. Should you feel you want to get a stone for each chakra then you could start with small, inexpensive tumbled pebbles and add to them as you go along, as you wish. It isn't essential.

Buying crystals can be great fun and can do a lot for your energy level. The general rule is that you allow the crystal to choose you rather than the other way round. Just put out your hand over the collection of crystals and wait a second until you feel that you know which one to pick up. That one's yours. You then have a responsibility to take care of it so it can do its best for you.

Keeping it clean is very important since it works by both absorbing and giving out energy. Your quartz watch keeps perfect time because the tiny crystal emits a regular stream of electrons. Having chosen your crystal, steep it overnight in a solution of sea salt and water, then rinse it and pat it dry with some clean kitchen paper before putting it wherever you are going to keep it. It's not a good idea to have clear quartz in your bedroom since if you are sensitive, its energy may keep you awake. Amethyst would be better for its calming effect.

If your crystals have been working hard they can become less effective unless you re-energize them regularly. Some therapists will keep them in a bed of salt, others wash them regularly in sea salt solution or even return them to the earth for a while. I put mine in the soil around my plants (and sometimes forget them!), or sometimes at the base of trees in my garden. I re-energize them regularly by putting them in sea salt and water and leaving them outside during the night of the full moon. Every now and then I feel that one of them needs to return to the earth permanently and I take it somewhere special and, with a little ceremony of gratitude for all its work, give it back to the earth.

If you decide to choose a crystal for each chakra, then I've recommended a selection in each chapter. One for each chakra is enough, but I have no doubt that once you make a relationship with crystals, you'll want to add to your collection.

Water

Always have a glass of water to drink at the end of exercises and meditations. I use energized water which I make by leaving a quartz crystal in the jug of my water filter. Sometimes I also charge water with color by placing it in the appropriate colored bottle with the crystal whose energy I particularly want at that moment and leaving it in sunlight to charge. Try it—you'll be surprised at how it can shift your energy.

Comfort List

Making a comfort list is a good thing to do before you begin. There'll be times when you need to gently take care of yourself (ideally all the time). Until you get used to doing that as a matter of course, a list of things that make you feel good will help you. Stick a copy of it on your fridge door, in your office desk, by the bed and, of course, have a copy in your safe place.

As you go along and get more in touch with your whole self, you'll know what you need and may then rearrange your list according to the chakra you're wanting to nurture. The exercises in the following chapters will give you an indication of what would be helpful. But, for now, just start a list that you can then improve upon. My list includes

- walking in my garden or on the beach
- collecting shells, leaves and other pretty things
- standing in the shower for a long time feeling the water cleansing not only my body but my aura too, or having a long luxurious bath in perfumed water

- swimming
- dancing—I like dancing alone in my home, sometimes just moving to the music with my eyes closed
- riding my bicycle
- having a hug
- talking with my friends
- listening to the silence
- listening to the wind-chimes
- washing and rearranging my crystals
- lighting candles to increase their sparkle
- playing some lovely music
- being in the garden at dawn and watching the first rays of the sun
- meditating and feeling the joy of transcending—this is more than comfort: it is euphoric, ecstatic and beyond description
- making love
- having a massage
- curling up with a book
- spending time in a bookshop or library

And so it goes on.

I'm sure, if you let your mind wander, you can make your own list. Enjoy yourself making it, and use it whenever you want to. Turn to it when you feel bored, if you want to nibble and you know you're not really hungry or if things just feel a bit heavy and you need to relax and change the pace.

Being able to change your internal energy when necessary is very important and often you can do this quite simply by doing something to nurture yourself, with almost instantaneous results. When I'm working on myself, I use all the elements—fire, earth, air and water—

EQUIPMENT CHECK LIST

- *The 7 Healing Chakras*
- Two exercise books
- Angel cards
- Tape recorder
- Small place reserved for your spiritual work
- Candles
- Crystals
- Pen
- Glass of water
- Comfort list

---

in some form to cleanse my space and make it sacred. I'll talk more of this in Chapters 4–7 since each of the first four chakras is associated with one of these elements.

When I do workshops, I take all my singing bowls, bells and gongs, incense, etc. with me (much to the consternation of airport officials) to keep the energy clean and fine where we're working, to dissipate pain and to promote healing.

Questionnaire

Now you're all set to begin. Before you do so, take a little time to complete this questionnaire. It'll only take a few minutes, but you might be surprised at what you find:

Root Chakra

(a) Do you feel, or have you ever felt that you don't really belong anywhere or that you're lonely wherever you are?

(b) Do you feel that you want to escape from your life, for example by drinking, taking drugs, having out-of-body experiences, committing suicide?

(c) Do you feel ambivalent about life and sometimes wish you were dead?

(d) Do you feel disappointed in sex, are impotent (unless this is associated with some physical illness) or fail to have real orgasms?

(e) Did you have some trauma, distress or difficulty between conception and the age of three to five?

(f) Do you feel insecure and perhaps need to compensate for that feeling, for example by hoarding, by indulging in buying things you don't really need or refusing to spend your money?

(g) Are you low in energy and often feel weak, tired or sick?

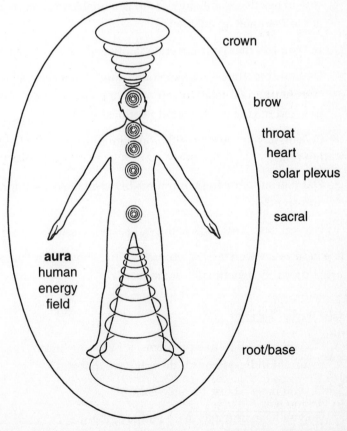

Figure 1: The Chakra System

(h) Do you have physical problems in your legs or feet, or suffer from hemorrhoids or chronic constipation?

If you answer "yes" to most of the above then you may well have some problem with your root chakra.

Sacral Chakra

(a) Do you have difficulty with your sexuality or with the giving or receiving of sexual pleasure, sometimes feeling either frozen or aggressive?

(b) Do you have difficulty with being gently touched and nurtured?

(c) Is your sex drive quite low or are you unable to achieve orgasm or get or maintain an erection?

(d) Do you feel that your general vitality and stamina are low?

(e) Do you sometimes channel your sexual desire into fantasy rather than have a real relationship or have many sexual partners so as to avoid having a committed relationship?

(f) Do you have problems with your kidneys, bladder or with retaining fluid?

(g) Did you suffer distress or trauma between the ages of three to five and eight?

(h) Do you have problems with your sense of taste?

If you have answered "yes" to most of the above, your sacral chakra could probably benefit from some work.

Solar Plexus Chakra

(a) Do you have digestive problems, for example ulcers, heartburn or recurrent indigestion? Or do you have diabetes?

(b) Do you have a fiery, irritable nature?

(c) Do you have difficulty with authority figures, either feeling small and insignificant or aggressive and rebellious?

(d) Do you feel anger or rage that erupts now and then (maybe after using alcohol) and that you have difficulty in accessing at other times?

(e) Did you suffer distress or trauma between the ages of eight and twelve?

(f) Do you sometimes feel powerless or sometimes so powerful that it frightens you?

(g) Have you had difficulty in achieving your potential no matter how hard you work?

(h) Do you have a problem with will—either being weak-willed, often going along with the opinions of others rather than forming your own? or being willful and going your own way regardless of the effects of your actions on other people?

"Yes" to most of these means that your personal power, prosperity and will could be enhanced by clearing your solar plexus.

Heart Chakra

(a) Do you find it difficult to love or feel loved?

(b) Are you negative and pessimistic, or bossy and dictatorial?

(c) Do you get involved in other people's lives and find it difficult to step back and let them make their own mistakes?

(d) Do you feel exhausted, fatigued or drained much of the time?

(e) Do you have problems with your heart, blood pressure or circulation, or have asthma or respiratory problems?

(f) Are you impatient and intolerant, or so patient and tolerant that people take advantage of you?

(g) Did you suffer distress and trauma between the ages of twelve and fifteen or sixteen?

(h) Do you have difficulty feeling forgiveness, compassion or empathy, or feel so compassionate and empathic that you are dragged down by other people's pain?

If you answer "yes" to most of the above then you have a problem with your heart chakra. Though for most chakras the problem is usually that there is a block, with the heart chakra it is just as likely that it is stuck open, leaving you vulnerable to all that's going on around you.

This is a problem suffered by many healers and others in caring professions. It's what leads to burnout. Learning to close down the chakras when necessary is just as important as keeping them free and open (see Protection exercises on page 57).

Throat Chakra

(a) Do you have difficulty with your hearing or speech?

(b) Do you often find yourself being misunderstood or are you aware that you have difficulty in expressing yourself?

(c) Have you had difficulty finding your true path, career or vocation?

(d) Have you had problems with your thyroid, your throat, your ears or your neck?

(e) Did you suffer any distress or trauma between the ages of fifteen or sixteen and twenty to twenty-one?

(f) Do you feel that your creativity is blocked or that you are not a creative person?

(g) Do you have difficulty with any of the rhythmical functions in your life, for example the rhythm of your breathing, your heartbeat, your menstrual cycle, or keeping time with the beat of music or in dancing?

(h) Do you have any difficulty with communication, including being able to listen attentively to other people's point of view?

Not only your communication but your creativity and your vocation can be clarified by work at your throat chakra. If you answered "yes" to most of these questions, you have some difficulty here.

Brow Chakra

(a) Do you suffer from migraine or other headaches?

(b) Do you have difficulty with internal regulation of some kind—for example hormonal, temperature, mood, violence?

(c) Do you have nightmares?

(d) Are you unable to visualize your future?

(e) Do you have difficulty with insight either into your own problems or those of other people?

(f) Do you feel stuck and in need of liberation and freedom?

(g) Do you feel guilty that in spite of all the things you have, you're still not happy?

(h) Did you suffer distress or trauma between the ages of twenty-one and twenty-six?

As we reach this level, the problem is often more one of lack of development than a block, though blocks do occur. A "yes" answer to most of the above would indicate that you could use some work here. Opening this chakra makes available possibilities you may hardly have dreamed of. Please note that it is usual for this chakra to develop only in your twenties, so do allow yourself time if you're still younger than that.

Crown Chakra

(a) Do you have a sense of being called to do healing, channeling or becoming involved in some mystical art?

(b) Do you wish to be more enlightened and have a sense of oneness with all things?

(c) Do you have a feeling of bliss, wholeness or euphoria not induced by anything external (for example drugs, or being in love), even if only for fleeting moments?

(d) Do you wish to be able to see beyond the material and see all of life as a wonderful opportunity to learn?

(e) Do you feel flooded with love for all things?

(f) Do you feel a wish to have a direct connection with God, the universe or whatever you call the great force?

(g) Are you able to see those who have hurt or abused you with compassion, forgiveness and even gratitude for the teaching they gave you?

(h) Can you view life with joy and unending love?

If you can answer "yes" to most of the above then you are well on your way to living in harmony and balance and to clearing much of the damage that you've suffered on your way to learning what you needed to learn in this lifetime. Within this state there's a responsibility, however. That is to share generously (though not obtrusively), to model a way of being to others who are on the path and to continue to strive for further enlightenment. At this point, life becomes much more joyful and easy, though there are still lessons to be learned as your journey continues.

I hope the journey, the "Rainbow Journey," to find your real self is exhilarating and filled with wonder. My heart and my love go out to you as you begin.

A SYMPATHETIC EAR

As you start your "rainbow journey," if you aren't in therapy, it would be good for you to try to bring to mind someone with whom you can talk if need be. There'll be times when you're confronted by things from the past that you don't really like or want to remember. Please, at those times, bear in mind that you have already survived. Nothing from the past can really hurt you now. It's over. What remains are the feelings you shut away. If you're aware that there are some really painful memories there, now would be a good time to look for a compassionate therapist. (You may find that the right therapist will just appear in your life. As you move along and learn to trust the universe and what it offers you, you'll become good at looking at each opportunity that arises.)

THREE

The Basics of Spirituality

∽

Before we begin work, let's clarify some of the concepts we'll be using. As with any subject, we need to begin with the basics, to define them and their relationship to each other. Perhaps this is even more important when dealing with something as wonderful as spirituality and healing which have almost defied definition despite being so real. Although people have been aware of their spirituality for centuries, describing it, let alone proving it, has been difficult until comparatively recently.

So what then is spirituality? Well, I suppose it feels different to each person. I can share with you how it feels to me:

> Spirituality is a river. A river of clear sparkling conscious-
> ness. A stream of light. My connection with God. My
> connection with the whole universe. It flows into me and
> around me, is part of me, fills every bit of me. It brings me
> calm and peace, joy and wisdom and amazing energy. It
> simultaneously slows me and suspends me in time and yet
> enlivens everything. It gives me clarity and enhances speed
> of thought and action while attenuating time. It sends me a
> steady stream of ideas—ready-formed knowings—and all
> accompanied by a glowing, exhilarating sense of serenity.
> So clear, so natural, so extraordinarily ordinary.

Though some personal effort, dedication and motivation were required on my part to clear the way and open the connection with my soul, since I learned to do this the energy has continued to flow so easily, so fluidly, so wonderfully. It is my natural state of being, it feels complete, perfect. All I have to do is ask. Ask and prepare—the rest is easy: like opening a tap—the water flows. And when it starts to happen it feels like a stream gently flowing—then sometimes flowing so fast that I can hardly keep up with it. There may be a patch so slow moving I might think it had stopped except for the feeling that's still there—excitement, exhilaration, crystal clarity, total awareness as though I'm almost standing aside while the stream of energy rushes through. Suddenly the pace changes again. Sometimes I want to cry, my breathing almost ceasing—little breaths maintaining my body as the God-energy uses me as a vehicle through which to flow. I stand aside and watch the miracle happen. Watch the wonderful light. Listen to the stream of thought. Hope, childlike, that it will continue and never stop. Feel grateful. Hardly dare move in case it stops, though I know it won't. Feel such reverence.

In the wonder, there is life, light, radiance and a feeling of being young, in tune, in touch, a gentle but definite power, wisdom, elation coursing through. And afterward there's a feeling of such joy, such peace. Sometimes there's a desire to be alone and quiet. At others, an urgent need to share, or to ground the love, to pass on the healing. And then the feeling of being grounded, healed, whole, joyful and healthy. This is my experience of my spirituality.

The spirit, or the soul, has been variously defined as that part of us which is essential to life and yet which has no tangible or visible substance; the immortal essence of our being; our higher self; or that part of us which has the functions of loving, thinking and willing. It is responsible for feats that are generally recognized as beyond the range of general human experience. Some would say it's the part of God that resides in us and joins us as a single body of humanity.

The soul has little to do with religion, though it's often in religion that those in pain or distress seek it. Sadly, religion often divides us, whereas spirituality always unites. Whatever the words you choose to describe the phenomenon of spirit, you can learn to be consciously aware of this aspect of yourself and to start to use it as a powerful tool that will make astounding changes in your life.

Our spirit is eternal; human experience but a moment. The whole is like a string of pearls—the thread being the spirit, while the pearls are lifetimes of earthly existence. Each is apparently complete, but in reality they are tiny parts of the whole everlasting essence of life. Nothing truly dies. Like trees that lie dormant in the winter, appear to come alive in the spring, blossom, lose their leaves and wait for the next spring, we too have our cycle. It is that unending spirit we can tap into now and use for our own benefit and that of others.

We're all spiritual beings, albeit at present human. Our spirituality is an ever-present factor in our daily lives. Some people actively recognize and utilize that part of themselves, whereas others haven't as yet done so. This book is intended to help you not only to recognize your spirit, but to mobilize it and begin to use it in every aspect of your life as you become healed, whole and healthy.

The Art of Healing

In places our river has become dammed with debris from the past, jammed with the flotsam and jetsam of life. We need to treat ourselves gently as we dislodge some of the wreckage and disentangle ourselves from the past. We must sensitively shake ourselves free of the feelings, hurts and bitterness that have clogged our natural flow and cut us off from the love, both human and divine, that nurtures us— our spiritual chicken soup. Healing enables us to free ourselves, get in balance and return to wholeness.

Healing is an art whereby what is unhealthy, dis-eased, compromised or unwell is returned to its natural state of health and well-being. Basically, it's about love. In whatever form it takes, healing always empowers, encouraging our consciousness to take responsibility for the well-being of the whole.

Whatever the illness, studies have proven that the psychological state of the person is of prime importance in the process of recovery. And since our psychological state is dependent upon our peace of mind which, in turn, is a function of our spirit, so the recovery from illness always involves a spiritual process. Essentially, the body cannot heal without being in balance with the mind and the spirit, nor can healing occur in the absence of love.

Although acts of healing are reported in both the Old and New Testaments of the Bible as well as in other ancient and religious writings, they're not simply a thing of the past. In the 20th century, healings still take place all over the world every day—in churches, in synagogues and other holy places, in doctors' offices, consulting rooms, by the roadside at accidents and in many other places. The mother who holds her sick baby and allows her love to flow into the child is aiding its recovery even though medical help may also be required.

There are doctors who pray for their patients, and surgeons who pray before going into the operating room. There are those who work specifically as healers in their own homes and in practices around the world. In every culture, there are shamans who ask for divine intervention for themselves and others. In fact, healing occurs wherever anyone has the love and faith to call to some power of goodness beyond themselves for help.

How Does It Work?

Healing occurs by the transmission of energy from a divine source to the recipient via a healer who simply acts as a conduit. The healer takes little real part in the transaction, except to prepare a safe and loving atmosphere for the healing to take place and to be as perfect a tool as possible. I sometimes try to explain it using the analogy of starting a car with a dead battery by using jumper cables. The healer transfers the initial boost of energy to get you started but you must then do your part by keeping the engine running.

Just as electricity can be measured, so the energy which passes from the healer can be recorded in terms of its electromagnetic and electrostatic properties and can be photographed by means of Kirlian photography. Healing has been well researched and proven. Indeed the research alone is the topic of a four-volume study by Dr. Daniel Benor, *Healing Research—Holistic Energy Medicine and Spirituality.*

Healing can take place through the "laying on of hands," through prayer, either formally or in a religious setting or simply by a spontaneous plea, or can be performed by flowing energy through the chakras without the healer ever having touched the patient at all.

The degree of healing is governed by what's right at that moment. For some, there'll be a spontaneous "miracle" with total remission of illness, although more usually it's a much more gradual process. For others, there may be simply a sense of peace. Healing when someone's dying won't reverse the cause of death but may allow all concerned, the recipient and the family and friends, to have a sense of peace and dignity as the person passes back to the spiritual world.

Though healing is still ridiculed by many and denied by even more, those who have actually approached it with an open mind (and many skeptics also) have felt, if not its power, then its peace. However, a word of caution. Though miracles do occur, beware of those who profess to perform them. Sadly, there are many who, from the point of view of their ego rather than from their spirit or their heart, profess to be able to perform miracles, leaving those in need feeling disappointed and disillusioned. Miracles are in the hands of God and not in the mind or control of humans. When we're privileged to be used as the tool for such powerful healing, there's a feeling of great humility and wonder rather than pride in the mind of the healer.

Absent Healing

Barbara Brennan describes in her book *Hands of Light* how, as early as the 12th century, the phenomenon of one person being able to affect another, even from a distance, was reported by Boirac and Liebeault. This phenomenon of distant, or absent, healing is a powerful tool which is still used by many healers today. Most healers have a list of those who have asked for healing, and spend some time each day focusing loving, healing energy toward those people, and also to troubled areas in the world.

This is something you can join in, too. Perhaps the most useful way is to send out the thought, with as much love as you can muster, that healing will be given where it's needed most. Some individuals who are strongly opposed to the concept of healing would not wish to receive, and it's essential to respect this. Sending out healing to those who don't wish to have it is a form of assault and should be avoided. To send out love to the planet with a pure heart and our highest integrity, with the intention that this will go to heal wherever it's needed most, is a different matter and I know that the healing is then directed by a higher wisdom.

However, this is a book about self-healing; the love and energy we use to heal others can also be used to help ourselves. Although very often we do need someone or something outside ourselves, be it a doctor, practitioner, medication or practical help, we can do much to heal ourselves. The power is yours. You can learn to clear your energy, access your spirituality and mobilize your innate power to heal yourself. For many, our innate ability to heal ourselves seems to be lost as we abdicate responsibility for our well-being to doctors, friends, counselors, the church or anyone else who's willing to take it. In doing so, we as individuals, families, societies, social groups, nations and the planet have lost the harmony and balance that was originally the common order of the universe. Undoubtedly, this was the path we were meant to take in order to learn that we need to return to the basics: love, healing, integrity, mutual support, honesty. It is there that we shall have all we need and more.

I'm not suggesting we let go of the modern ways of healing, nor that you stop any kind of help you're currently undergoing. Within the healing sphere, there's often a place for medication to relieve suffering and prevent untimely death, for example from infections. Modern medicine does, however, need to be accompanied by spiritual gifts and qualities if it's to achieve the best possible results. Mostly, the power and responsibility of the "patient" for his or her welfare needs to be harnessed and utilized.

Attempts have certainly been made over the last twenty years to help medical students see their patients as people rather than as "cases" and there's been a move toward helping patients be more involved in their own care. Sadly, however, there's still sometimes a tendency to see the person as "the gall bladder in bed ten" and the doctor as the god who can cure everything. This isn't only the fault of the medical profession. As I said earlier, there's often a desire on the part of the person who's unwell or unhappy to get someone else to do the work for them. True healing cannot occur in that way.

My personal crusade has been to marry orthodox medicine with healing and complementary therapies. This integrated, truly holistic approach can address each of us as a whole being—physically, emotionally, mentally and spiritually. This, I believe, is the only sensible way forward. Attempting to continue to separate the ancient from the modern, the spiritual from the physical, is like trying to hold back the tide.

The Right Time, the Right Place

No matter how you may try to avoid the real problem, hide the real pain or control the situation, in the end, healing takes place where and when it's needed.

Some years ago, a woman came to see me complaining of a bad back. She could hardly walk when she came into my consulting room and had to be helped onto the couch. As we started to talk it was obvious to me that although the problem she complained of was acute physical pain and lack of function, her real problem was within her marriage and with the childhood difficulties that had prompted her to choose an abusive relationship. I told her that although I was happy to do what I could for the pain, what she really needed to do was to come for some psychotherapy and sort out why she was allowing herself to be in such an abusive situation. She had some healing and walked out of my room standing up straight and pain free. She made a further appointment for a full assessment for psychotherapy but never kept it.

I didn't hear from her for almost two years until she returned again with a similar complaint of acute back pain. Once again, she was almost unable to walk. We talked about her current circumstances and, in particular, her marriage, which had continued to be mutually abusive. On this occasion she was at the point where she was more available to some psychological input. When she walked out of my room that day, once more totally free of physical pain, she made a series of appointments and began the work necessary to change her life. She did this very successfully with a combination of healing and psychotherapy. Her back hasn't troubled her in the last eight years and she and her husband are still in their marriage, though they've long since ceased to abuse each other.

Much of the healing work was to correct the energy blocks she'd developed over years of abuse from childhood up to the time she eventually decided to take responsibility and get well. She had tried to abdicate responsibility for her wellness to everyone, including me. She'd had surgical procedures, analgesic medication and much input from her general practitioner, but she was unable to utilize their excellent care without removing the energy blocks that were rendering her physically stuck. Severe back pain was the final result of her failure to heed the messages on both the spiritual and emotional level that all wasn't well.

The Etheric Bodies

The human body is, in the main, so dense that we can see, touch, smell and feel it. The part that most of us cannot readily see—the aura and, within it, the chakras (described in detail later in this chapter)—is termed the etheric body, or more accurately, bodies. Every living thing emits an energy field and the human energy field, or aura, is enlivened by the swirling, spinning streams of energy created by its constantly moving chakras. The chakras are to the aura what the currents are to the ocean: they transform it into a living and tremendous force.

It's through this extended part of the body that energy flows into the physical body to keep it vitalized and alive. This energy is as essential to our life and well-being as food and air. Without this life force, we couldn't survive. And just as the physical body is in a state of constant change, with cells forever in a cycle of regeneration and decay, so the etheric part of our body is in a state of constant movement. It swirls around us, transferring energy into and out of the physical body. It senses what's around us and acts as the repository of thought forms and memory.

The aura gives us essential information that fills the gap between the physical and the psychological, between biology and mysticism, physical medicine and psychotherapy. The aura is the place where thoughts and emotions are located as real substance, where the forms of thought and emotion passing between people as we interact can actually be seen. The substance appears to those who can see it like mucus or smoke or flashing light.

Everything about you—from your stamina, endurance, the texture of your skin and the shine of your hair to your perception of a beautiful sunset, your enjoyment of a day in a forest or your delight at seeing someone do well—can be affected by improving your energy system. You can do this by cleansing, balancing and nurturing your chakras and consequently surrounding yourself with a peaceful and healthy aura.

The aura, which is really a subtle extension of the physical body, is clearly visible to some people. It consists of a series of seven layers of varying thickness and color, each associated with one of the chakras and each with a specific function. Sometimes the sense of individual layers may be lost, the whole blending into a shining, shimmering, ever-moving mass of colored light.

The ability to see the aura is simply an extension of normal vision. It's a capacity readily available to some and as normal as seeing a friend's face is to the rest of us. Those who have the power to see the more subtle energy fields are simply more sensitive to a broader range of vibrations than is common. Those who can't perceive the aura are often disbelieving and prone to ridiculing those who can, and so an important contribution to the development of new tools for understanding the human condition has often been ignored. As a consequence, we're moving more slowly toward a more universal state of peace and harmony than we might otherwise. Most children have the capacity to see the aura and often the individual chakras within it, but they usually lose this ability at a very early age unless it's nurtured. A friend of mine told me excitedly that her child had brought home a drawing from nursery school in which she'd depicted her mother apparently with ribbons flowing from her hair. The child explained that these were Mummy's "colored bits" and described perfectly the aura as she saw it.

Most of us even by nursery school age have forgotten who we really are, our skills as ancient wise spirits being forgotten too. Although these can be rediscovered in later life by doing the necessary spiritual work, they're virtually lost to those who, for one reason or another, don't want to use them or are threatened by the fact that others appear to have powers that they themselves lack.

Even if you dispute the existence of the aura (see Appendix B, page 226) for information on proof of etheric bodies), you may admit to feeling a presence around some people. Most who have been in the presence of Mother Teresa or Mother Meera or other powerful healers or mystics couldn't help but be aware of some tangible force that surrounds them. Their very powerful and highly developed aura makes it difficult to miss.

The same phenomenon is present around each and every one of us. To achieve such brilliance we need to work on clearing blockages and the psychological and emotional debris that has clogged our flow of energy and prevented us from fulfilling our potential.

Similarly, from time to time, you may have encountered someone who has a disturbed aura, which can be as palpable as the clear bright presence. And just as one who is highly evolved can heal others with the healing energy they emanate, so those who are disturbed can unwittingly affect us also. Learning to protect ourselves is essential and before we begin any aura work we'll look at Protection Exercises (see page 57).

I cannot emphasize strongly enough the good sense of learning to protect your own energy against contamination by others and against allowing it to be drained by those who, in their desperation, feed off the energy of more healthy souls. Despite the fact that I'm very aware of the dangers of not protecting myself, there have been a couple of occasions when I've failed to respect this aspect of my work and have allowed myself to be hurt by the energy that's arisen while working with people who, through no fault of their own, have been involved in unwholesome practices.

It's quite arrogant to believe that we're powerful enough to overcome or withstand such negative forces. The power of love and good is always superior to that of evil, but we should have a healthy respect for both. Just as it would be foolhardy to walk out into the middle of a busy street assuming that God will protect us, it's foolish not to take adequate precautions in the face of possible danger.

As a healer and as a psychiatrist, it's inevitable that I deal with a lot of pain, and without the protection exercise I would become burnt out and of little value to anyone.

There's nothing in this book that will harm you in any way, but there may be those in your sphere who have suffered much and who carry with them in their aura not only the emotional and spiritual scars of their abuse, but also negativity that you could certainly do without. Our aim is to free ourselves in order to be healthy and happy and then to flow love and healing energy out into the world. Our aim is not to pick up anything unhealthy from elsewhere. Sometimes in their naivety and overzealous wish to help, novices to spiritual work can pick up pain and damage and pass it on to others.

The Energy of Life

Most cultures have their own term for the life force or energy that is essential to our very existence, let alone our well- being. Whether this is the *chi* of Chinese medicine or *prana* of Indian teaching, the energy referred to is the same. It's the force that is the basic constituent of life, and the same energy that becomes visible in the aura.

While physical food sustains the life of the physical body, this spiritual energy is essential to nurture us and lift us beyond a merely physical form. It is this energy—spiritual energy—that accounts for our higher feelings: our capacity for clarity, courage, charity, endeavor, love, loyalty, faith. It is this energy that, at times, renders us capable of more than our mere physical bodies could possibly achieve. It is the stuff of our soul.

Occasionally you may have had the experience of suddenly being aware that someone is looking at you even though you can't see them directly. Or perhaps you've been in the position where someone has been standing just too close and you feel invaded. Perhaps someone has stepped a little closer and, almost against your will, you took a step backwards. Your aura and, in particular, your chakras are acting as an early warning system and are protecting that area of personal space around you. This "space" is your aura, which is filled with energy, rather like an egg surrounding you. It is in intimate contact with you and affects (and is affected by) every thought, word, feeling and memory that you have.

It's actually part of you. It's part of your body, an extension of you, so much so that if you should lose part of your physical body, for example by amputation, the aura of that part still remains—the phantom limb which has been studied so widely. The only difference between your aura and what you usually think of as your body is that your aura consists of pure energy, which is normally invisible to the eye, not dense enough to touch in our usual understanding of touch, and from which we have no physical sensations. For example, you don't sense pain when your aura touches the sharp corner of your desk, but you do when your physical body bumps into it. That makes it no less real, however. Neither wind, nor electricity, nor radio waves are visible to the human eye, but few people these days would deny their existence.

Damage to the aura can also be seen. For example, cocaine use can cause holes in the aura and the energy that flows in through these holes can be extremely damaging to all levels—physical, emotional, mental and spiritual. People who are using illicit drugs often do so in quite sordid surroundings in an unwholesome atmosphere with other people who are sick. It's no wonder that they may develop disturbed behavior that can continue for long periods of time, sometimes even years, after the drug abuse has discontinued. Without proper cleansing and attention to the chakras and healing of the aura, some of these people never fully recover—they continue to struggle with a variety of problems that appear unrelated to their past drug misuse. If we add to this the fact that some therapy never really confronts the underlying issues (including spiritual), it's small wonder that many will return again and again to their drug of choice to get some meager comfort in what they perceive as an otherwise hostile environment.

The Chakras

The word *chakra* is Sanskrit, meaning wheel, and refers to the many vortices of energy that penetrate not only the aura but the physical body as well. There are seven major, twenty-one minor and many lesser chakras. Others are being revealed through time. Of the lesser chakras, the most commonly used are those found in the palms of the hands and the soles of the feet.

To most, the chakras are more readily felt than seen. The easiest way to sense them is to hold the hand a few inches away from the physical body. The presence of clothing doesn't impede the energy or the ease with which it can be felt, so it's rarely necessary to remove any clothing to receive healing.

If you hold your hands in front of you, palms facing each other about eight inches apart, and bring them very gently and slowly toward each other, you can feel a subtle change, rather like a soft cushion, as the aura of one hand meets that of the other. Why not play with this concept and have some fun discovering this new aspect of you? The chakras are so sensitive that they are affected not only by the energy of other people but also by the energy that hangs around in some places. We've already ascertained that you feel good in the presence of some people whereas others drain you. This feeling may arise with someone you've never met before and yet suddenly, on being in the same room with them, you feel at peace. Similarly, you may come into contact with another person for only a few minutes and feel uncomfortable, even ill, and yet there appears to be no real reason for this. We all use various energetic tactics to protect ourselves, to manipulate others and to hide our vulnerability, though often we may be unaware of this on a conscious level.

Though we can learn to protect ourselves from outside influence to a large degree, what we really need to do is to build up a healthy system that keeps us flexible on all levels—physical, emotional, mental and spiritual.

To achieve this, each chapter of *The Seven Healing Chakras* will take you through a specific chakra looking at its functions, its characteristics, and the kinds of problems that develop if we have a "block." The exercises to help clear these blocks and meditations will prompt spiritual growth. Ultimately, your whole system will become more healthy and flexible.

Although the healthy functioning of our chakra system is essential to our positive well-being, just as some people survive with digestive systems that are clogged and sluggish, leaving them feeling constantly under par, so the majority of us survive with disturbed and distorted chakras. Though it's not likely to kill us (directly at least), a reduced energy flow leaves us feeling never as well as we might, lacking sparkle and joy.

The Chakra System

The specific location of each chakra is discussed in greater detail in the chapter dedicated to it (see Figure 1 page 29). However, it's useful here to look at the system as a whole. Chakras appear like spinning wheels of light. When healthy, they spin in a clockwise direction, drawing in energy from the universal energy field to continually revitalize our whole being. Since they spin at different speeds, each emits a different light frequency, which is seen as a different color. The lowest or base (root) chakra is red, and the others bear the other colors of the spectrum—orange, yellow, green, blue, indigo or purple and finally white.

Each of the major chakras is associated with one of the seven layers of the aura. The first chakra is associated with the layer closest to the physical body, the second next to this and so on. Although theoretically each of these takes the color of the chakra that governs it, in practice this is rarely the case. In fact, the aura is more often seen as one single color—often yellow; more commonly, it will have areas of dense color within it, the distinct layers appearing to be fused. Sometimes the layers are obscured by other elements—for example by old emotion or old thought forms. Unresolved emotions such as unexpressed anger may stay in the aura for years.

Although they are always numbered from the base up, the major chakras have been given different names by different schools, which can cause confusion. Some use names associated with their location and others with their function. For the purposes of this book, the seven chakras we'll be focusing on are labeled as follows:

CHAKRA 1—BASE OR ROOT CHAKRA

This chakra is situated at the base of the spine, between the coccyx and the pelvic bone and its color is red. Its main function is to keep us grounded in the physical world and to keep us alive. It's associated with physical sensation. The first layer of the aura is similarly associated with the physical.

CHAKRA 2—SACRAL CHAKRA

This chakra is to be found in the midline below the navel. Its color is orange and its main function is related to reproduction and the giving and receiving of sexual pleasure. The second layer of the aura is similarly associated with the emotional.

CHAKRA 3—SOLAR PLEXUS CHAKRA

The solar plexus is situated either in the midline or slightly to the left above the stomach. Its color is yellow. This is the site where we form opinion. Here is the center of potency, power and will. The third layer of the aura is associated with mental functions.

CHAKRA 4—HEART CHAKRA

This is sometimes referred to as a transitional chakra since the lower three are concerned with the physical and emotional and now we begin to move toward the spiritual. The heart bridges the two realms and is the center for human love. It's also a center for feeling and its color is emerald green. Its layer is the astral plane.

CHAKRA 5—THROAT CHAKRA

As its name implies, this chakra lies at the throat and is part of the realm of the divine. The throat chakra when well developed allows us to speak our truth with courage and also to listen and not judge. It's the home of our integrity and our vocation. Its color is blue or turquoise. The fifth layer is the etheric body.

CHAKRA 6—BROW CHAKRA (SOMETIMES ERRONEOUSLY REFERRED TO AS THE THIRD EYE)

This takes us up into the celestial and into love that surpasses human love. It is the site of clear vision in the spiritual sense. The layer associated with this chakra is the celestial body. Its color is purple or deep blue.

CHAKRA 7—CROWN CHAKRA

Situated at the top of the head, the crown chakra is our access to the divine, the spiritual realms. It allows us to draw in spiritual energy for our own use or to use to help others in healing. It is also the center of knowing—knowing without thought or reason. Here the whole is integrated: the physical, emotional, intellectual and spiritual.

The minor chakras are found

- at the front of each ear
- above each breast
- in the palm of each hand
- the sole of each foot

- behind each eye
- over the ovaries and testicles
- behind each knee

There are also chakras connected to the stomach and the thymus, one below the throat chakra, above the breast bone (sternum) between the two collarbones, at the major solar plexus chakra, and two are situated at the spleen. The lesser ones are commonly found at the site of joints and generally correspond to the sites of acupuncture points.

The major chakras at the sacrum, solar plexus, heart, throat and brow can be perceived at both the front and back of the body, though generally at a slightly higher level at the back (see Figure 2). They're con-

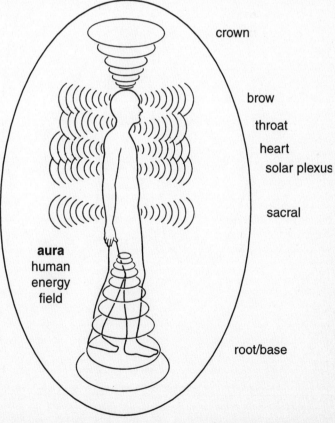

crown

brow

throat

heart

solar plexus

sacral

aura
human
energy
field

root/base

Figure 2: The Chakra System

nected centrally at the spinal column and ideally there should be a free flow of energy from front to back and back to front. The crown and base form a vertical axis that runs through the center of all the other chakras. It can be felt above the head, and forms a funnel of energy extending down from the base of the spine between the legs toward the ground.

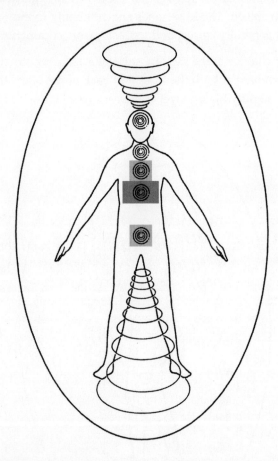

Figure 3: Major block at solar plexus with old bitterness, anger and pain prevents free flow of energy with development of secondary blocks elsewhere. The heart is incapable of true loving and the sacrum is unable to enjoy complete sexual release. Creativity and potential are restricted, as are open communication, vision and awareness.

Energy flows in both directions. The root chakra takes in energy from the earth and also allows us to ground spiritual energy much as a lightning rod grounds electricity. It gives us stability. Meanwhile, the crown chakra brings in energy from above and forms our direct access point for higher spiritual energy. The channel for the flow of energy between the crown and root is sometimes referred to as the vertical or central power current or channel. This intimate connection and inter-dependence means it's impossible to think of them in isolation when discussing their effect upon our total functioning as human beings.

Energy Blocks

Although a block is the term commonly used when a chakra is not functioning well, it covers a variety of difficulties. The chakra may be spinning too slowly, in the wrong direction, be hardly spinning at all (sometimes termed "silent"); it may be out of balance or indeed it may actually be damaged. It may be too active and brittle so that it can't gently open and close at your will. (See Figure 3.)

When a chakra is "open" (though they're never completely closed), there's little choice but to deal with the energy and the associated psychological material that's flowing through it. Although it's true that, to some extent, the greater the energy flow, the healthier we are, some of the energy we have to deal with can cause psychological or emotional pain. It's for this reason that we shut down or "block" our chakras in the first place.

These blocks are not there by accident. They're designed by you and put in place to protect you from what, at the time, you're unable to process. However, most of the blocks become outdated, preventing further growth.

Clearing them is rather like a spring cleaning exercise (see Figure 4, page 54). We look at all the things we've accumulated and discard some of them. In the process, we may come across something very beautiful that we'd like to bring back into the light. However, first it must be dusted and polished or cleared of layers of tarnish. Cleansing your chakras is rather like this.

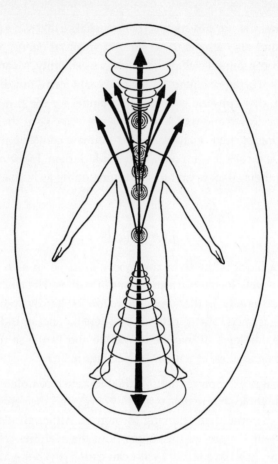

Figure 4: Release of old pain at the solar plexus allows for quick release of other chakras with increase in energy on all levels

Whatever the cause, your whole energy flow is affected by any disturbance. Since all the chakras are intimately linked, a block at one will affect the functioning of the others, causing physical, emotional and/or spiritual distress.

A reasonable analogy may be that if I have a blockage in a major vein in my leg, the circulation beyond the block will be affected by it. Though my body uses other channels to compensate and may appear to perform well in spite of the block, eventually the problem will become too severe to ignore and I'll need help to deal with it.

THE BASICS OF SPIRITUALITY 55

Similarly, and in very simple terms, if I have a block at my second chakra, there won't be adequate energy for optimal flow to the third, fourth, fifth, sixth or seventh. Even though each operates individually, the connection between them is essential for optimum efficiency.

Each of the major chakras is also associated with a major gland of the endocrine system and its dysfunction will therefore have far-reaching effects (see Appendix A, page 220). For example, since the throat chakra is associated with the thyroid gland and the thyroid gland has functions related to growth, motion, temperature control and much more, damage to or loss of function of the fifth chakra may have an impact on all of these functions.

Types of Block

Different types of energy block that correspond to psychological defense mechanisms serve different functions and we develop them to protect ourselves from what is too difficult to deal with at the time. They include

- the suppression of feelings, which typically leads to depression and despair (usually a heart chakra block)

- compression and compaction of rage which is perceived as potentially destructive if it's allowed to erupt (usually a solar plexus block)

- freezing of feelings, which often results in a lot of tension and a need to defend against any further possible attack (usually a heart chakra block)

- depletion of energy and abdication of power, which renders the person apparently helpless and in need of much support from others, hence protecting them from having to accept personal accountability and responsibility (solar plexus and/or sacral block)

- denial, which is usually a product of fear—here the person will often behave as though everything is fine while underneath there is chaos to such a degree that confronting it needs to be avoided at all costs to avoid possible breakdown (this can be present with a block at any chakra)

Many people use a combination of these blocks and move from one to another depending on the circumstances they find themselves in. All of us use blocks from time to time in order to regulate the flow of energy, depending on what we feel we can cope with. Sometimes these temporary blocks can be a very useful tool.

While consulting, I often move around in my chair—I move my hands, cross my legs, put an arm across my chest or touch my forehead as I move my energy—protecting and regulating the flow as I'm directed to. Most people do this quite unconsciously in what we've come to know as body language. In many cases, however, blocks become permanent structures, at worst, or habitual ways of damming the flow and avoiding certain aspects of ourselves, at best. All can be cleared and healed with time, gentleness and a genuine desire to do so. No one has a right to remove or attempt to dismantle any blocks you may have until they're invited by you to do so.

Coming into therapy implies the invitation to the therapist to do whatever is necessary to help you to get well. However, quite often I've found myself having to deal with the results of bungled therapy or incompetent attempts at healing. You are in charge, and though therapy is quite often a painful process, and there are, of necessity, things to be discussed that initially you may resist, if you find that something deep down tells you all is not well, heed that voice and at least discuss it with your therapist.

Our Work

The work you will be doing on yourself through *The Seven Healing Chakras* will be gentle and smooth. From time to time you'll have wonderful insights that will move you forward quite quickly, but you'll be constantly in control and can always proceed at your own pace.

But don't be surprised if progress is rapid. The aura can change in appearance quite quickly as work proceeds, and the clarity and spin of the chakras can be completely changed within one session of healing. However, you may be unable to sustain this new and intense inpouring of energy, so you might put the block back in place quite soon. Don't be discouraged by this: it's perfectly normal since, as with most intervention that produces lasting change, there needs to be a gradual development until a new way of being has been established. Just as a starving child may be unable to deal with a sudden feed of very rich milk, so the starving energy system may be unable to cope with a sudden blast of powerful energy.

One of the mistakes made by inexperienced but powerful healers is that they forget this. The sudden blasting through of blocks will lead the emotional and psychological material that caused the block to suddenly erupt into consciousness, and this can cause a healing crisis that the inexperienced healer is ill-equipped to deal with. All the work I recommend here will be gentle and will allow you to start to process repressed material in a very approachable way.

Protection Exercises

Some would say we should never protect ourselves since in doing so we acknowledge that there is something to fear. I don't subscribe to that. I feel we have a responsibility to keep our energy as pure as possible and to take care of it as we would anything else of value.

It's wonderful if we're in an environment where the energy is pure and we're with those who love us and surround us with positive energy so we can remain open, but for some people that's a rare occurrence. And when we have learned to recycle pain and neutralize it or allow angelic presences to dissipate it, we can do immense good by remaining open and cleansing energies wherever we are. People in our vicinity will feel the difference and respond positively to our presence.

However, until you reach that stage, please remember that if you are too open and unprotected it is all too easy to pick up what I call psychic junk from other people. We need to have a healthy respect for the work we're doing and for the fact that many people who are still stuck in their pain, especially emotional pain, are carrying around a heavy load of negative energy. Anger is particularly easy to pick up. It might be useful to think of anger as an iceberg—most of it is submerged but the rest projects outside. If anyone in your sphere uses drugs such as heroin, cocaine or amphetamines, there will often be aura damage that makes it easy to have negative energy stuck there. It will help neither them nor us if we allow it to be offloaded onto ourselves.

In any case, it's good practice to get into the habit of protecting yourself. Protecting ourselves means surrounding ourselves (and if you are a therapist, surrounding those with whom you work) with a shield of positive energy so that nothing negative can invade our space. Sometimes it also involves closing down our chakras while projecting round us energy that cannot be penetrated by others. There are several ways of doing this and eventually you will do it with a simple thought. But in the first place, please don't try to cut corners. Take your time to do it well.

Undoubtedly, the best protection is to constantly project a field of love around you—this acts as a coat of armor. With time, this is the method you may find yourself using. But this takes a lot of practice and sometimes, however well poised, we can be caught off balance and find our human side letting us down. I have to admit that, although I have used this method for years, on occasions, usually as a consequence of verbal abuse that touches some of my childhood pain, I haven't been quick enough to get other protection in place and have left myself open to picking up the other person's pain and anger and responding to it. So here are some other highly effective methods.

Method 1

Whenever you've finished working on yourself, or when you're going to be out and about in the world, especially if you're with one of those people who seems adept at draining your energy, take a few minutes to run through the following:

Take a couple of deep breaths and as you do so relax as much as you can. Imagine a beautiful white flower at the top of your head with its petals wide open. With a thought, see them close. Let the flower become a tight bud. Let your focus drop now to your brow. See there a beautiful deep blue or purple flower and, with a thought, allow its petals to close into a tight bud. Drop your focus now to your throat. See here a sky-blue or turquoise flower. Allow its petals to close and then allow your focus to drop to your heart. Here there is a beautiful green flower. Let its petals close also. Now to your solar plexus. Here there is a yellow flower. Let its petals close to a very, very tight bud. Now focus on your sacral chakra. Here is an orange flower. Let its petals close also. Your root chakra stays open to keep you constantly grounded and nourished by the earth. Cross your arms across your chest. Bow your head slightly. Now imagine that there is a beautiful midnight blue cloak beside you. Allow it to drape around you and over your head to fully protect you. Breathe. Know that you are protected.

Method 2

Take a couple of deep breaths and relax as much as you can. Imagine a beautiful white light streaming down above your head and spilling in a pyramid around you. Feel the pyramid become filled with light. Breathe it in and let it enter into every part of you so that you are filled

---

ACCEPTING SUPPORT

If you are currently having some emotional or psychological help, please do not stop it. Don't be tempted to stop medication or any other traditional intervention either. Discuss what you're doing and have some support system upon which you can call if you need it. But be aware that there are always people around who will rain on your parade. They may ridicule what you're doing and strangle the new and tender plant of your spiritual growth before it's had time to take root, so choose carefully who you confide in. Let your intuition guide you here. You do have intuition! Now's the time to get it out and use it. Your intuitive voice will generally lead you in a light and gentle way. As a general guide, if there is a voice saying in a parental way that you should do something, that is not your intuition but an internalized parent of long ago.

---

with and surrounded by light. Now, with a breath, cover the pyramid with pure golden light. Know that you carry it with you, that you can see and communicate through it, but that it will protect you from any in-flowing energy. Whenever it comes to mind to do so, reinforce it with more light.

Method 3

This is particularly useful for therapists and healers. Before you begin, cleanse your own energy field with an outward stream of love, breathing it out into your aura and sealing it with golden energy. Now, construct around you a column of light in which you can work. You may increase it to include your patient/client if you wish, but if you do so, be careful to ensure complete separation of your energies at the end of the session, sealing again your own energy and putting a protective coat separately around them before they leave. Know that you are protected.

So . . . let's move on to the first, the root chakra which is earthy, powerful and stabilizing and whose main desire is to keep us alive!

PART II

The Chakras

FOUR

The Root Chakra: The Crimson Base

∾

Spilled on this earth are all the joys of heaven.

—*Anonymous*

Have you ever wondered why some people have presence? Charisma? Why, whatever their circumstances, they're optimistic most of the time? Why they hardly ever appear to have a crisis of self-confidence and their self-esteem seems good? Some people seem to be able to manifest what they need and suffer a setback. Something always turns up for them. Is it luck? Astrological sign? Personality?

Well, maybe. But underlying all that is the fact that they're well grounded, have a good foundation, bonded well with their mothers or other primary caretakers, and have a good sense of their physical bodies. In fact, what they demonstrate is that they have a healthy, well-balanced, fast-spinning, unobstructed base chakra.

If you invest time and effort in nurturing the root chakra, you'll be richly rewarded in stability, security and a sense of belonging and self-esteem. Yet, because our daily lives today provide little real contact with the earth and very little time to nurture ourselves, these qualities often elude us. Even those with very stable beginnings can lose the feeling of inner security by neglecting or losing respect for their roots.

Without the strong, robust energy of this first chakra, our spiritual ascent is obstructed. In addition, we're unable to find true contentment or be healthy (either physically, emotionally or spiritually), and it's hard to find joy in being alive, let alone withstand the demands of life. If the root chakra is weak or closed, we feel lost, ungrounded. We drift like a leaf in the wind, seemingly without purpose, value or destination, and our self-esteem is poor.

So, survival is the name of the game. The root chakra aims to keep us alive no matter what. It governs our basic instincts—eating, sleeping, sex, self-preservation and conservation of the species. It's there to keep us going until we complete what we came here to do. It's associated with the adrenal glands (see Appendix A on endocrinological connections) and the fight or flight response that comes into play instinctively to protect us if we're under threat. It urges us to become all that we are capable of being, governing our drive to care for and nourish ourselves and to keep ourselves fit. In this way, we're ready not only to deal with whatever life sends our way but also to prosper. It assures us of the gift of good judgment, a tool necessary to avoid danger, while still allowing us to be adventurous and take risks.

From the earth arises not only our physical body and the food we eat, but also all the material goods we furnish our lives with. This chakra is about matter, substance, the earth and all that comes from it. It therefore relates to our eating patterns, how we take care of ourselves, our motivation to earn in order to live well, our ability to manifest what we need. It is the first of the seven major chakras, and if we do not ensure its stability and health it cannot ensure ours.

Though many seeking peace and spirituality attempt to discard the physical and concrete, believing that being materially minded is somehow anathema to being spiritual, little could be further from the truth. Certainly, to make an idol of material things is unhealthy, but we're here in a physical world, with physical bodies and needs for food, shelter, clothing and other creature comforts. Not only should we have them, but we should enjoy them.

We are spiritual beings trying our best to be human during this sojourn on the planet. My physical body is the visible evidence of my incarnation, and also the part of me that houses my spirit, my emotions and my intelligence. It interprets the physical world for me by use of its complex nervous system and senses. My body is, in fact, the means by which I work through whatever tasks I've set for myself in this lifetime. When we've taught all we have to teach, when we've learned all we came to learn, given all we have to give and received all we have to receive, then it will be time for us to depart and return to the freedom of the spirit. But, for the present, we're here and we must embrace the physical if we're not only to survive but to become the best we can be.

Building Good Foundations—Elementary Groundwork

Imagine you're building a house. Naturally, you begin by digging the foundations to ensure that there's a good strong base to support the structure. In some ways, the foundations are the most important part of a house. Without them, there's no way the house could survive the test of time or the impact of the elements. Our health and spiritual development need to have the same firm foundations.

Our root chakra is the first rung on the rainbow ladder and is equivalent to the foundations of a house that are dug deep down into the earth. If we skip the work at this stage and proceed to the higher—and for some, more exciting and attractive—chakras that govern our emotions, thoughts, vision and understanding, we do so at our peril. Without the fundamental groundwork, we cannot make truly satisfying headway that will support us through whatever difficult times may lie ahead. Without the cleansing and healing of the root chakra, we're ungrounded, with a flimsy attachment to the earth and, like a tree without roots, the first real storm will topple us.

This wonderful, robust chakra is the spring from which issues the fountain of energy that vitalizes everything as we proceed on our journey of enlightenment and discovery.

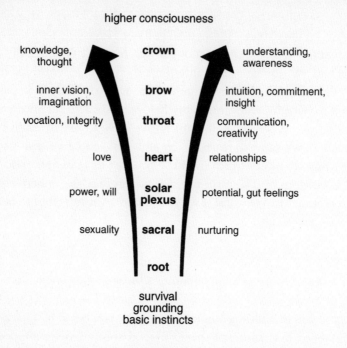

higher consciousness

	knowledge, thought	**crown**	understanding, awareness
	inner vision, imagination	**brow**	intuition, commitment, insight
	vocation, integrity	**throat**	communication, creativity
	love	**heart**	relationships
	power, will	**solar plexus**	potential, gut feelings
	sexuality	**sacral**	nurturing
		root	

survival
grounding
basic instincts

Figure 5: Clearing the root chakra allows the whole chakra system to open, with all the gifts that brings.

A Source of Energy

The root chakra is a wheel of light about three inches in diameter, which spins to form a funnel of light pointing toward the earth from the base of the spine or more accurately, the perineum (the piece of tissue between anus and vagina/scrotum). It's the slowest of all the chakras, spinning at the frequency of red light and thereby producing its distinct crimson color. The ruby gem emits light at the same frequency.

At the lower end of the central power channel, the root chakra affects all the others in a very powerful manner. It constantly maintains a flow of solid, grounding energy. It's also ready to send a surge of power up through all of the other chakras whenever necessary, as long as they're able to respond. Its effect on our vitality is crucial. Often, healing at this chakra improves your general energy and brings a new sense of balance and well-being. As your sense of security is improved, you'll experience less anxiety and improved sleep.

Work on any chakra brings improvements in every area of your life, but if you're not truly grounded the improvement can't be sustained—even if you feel better in the short term. Sometimes healers choose to work with the root chakra in order to help the patient become grounded, more stalwart and better able to deal with the rest of their difficulties. In this book's system of self-healing, I cannot overemphasize the value of cleansing and healing this chakra. It has the potential to shift all the other blocks in the system and to make work at the higher centers much easier. Being able to ground yourself at will is of the utmost importance (you will find an exercise to help you with this on page 78).

Well named, since it roots us to the planet, the root chakra gives us the opportunity to draw up the stimulating, dynamic energy of the earth. This connection also allows us to discharge anything negative which otherwise could cause stress and psychic overload. At the beginning of this chapter's meditations (see page 80), I suggest a gradual relaxation of the body with both feet flat on the floor and I ask that focus should be taken down through the physical body so that you can allow anything negative simply to flow out through the soles of the feet and the root chakra. In both meditations we use the root chakra's great gift of allowing us to regularly let go and return to the earth whatever is no longer needed, knowing it will be safely handled.

Discovering Our True Identity

The root chakra reminds us of who we truly are. It reminds us that we're part of the universe and prompts us to acknowledge our innate beauty and our unique worth and to recognize our oneness with creation. It gives us focus, discipline and a sturdy base from which to explore ourselves and the world. It prevents us from scattering our energies to the wind while it simplifies our existence and validates us as individuals with will and choice.

With a strong root chakra, we simply know that we're as amazing as all the other wonders of the universe and that we're just as essential to the overall plan. We fit into it as perfectly as the sunset, a waterfall or the deer in the forest. Irrespective of the way in which we contribute to the earth, we become aware that our contribution is essential and unique. Without any one of us, a shift would set in motion a chain of events that in some way would affect the delicate balance of all life. This knowledge gives us a pride in what we do and in doing it well. Whether we're mothering our children, working in a factory or being powerful executives, our performance is improved.

We also know that we are held in high esteem, as individuals, in a vast cosmos. It's no longer possible to view ourselves as insignificant little beings in a world that doesn't really need us. From a sense of the spirit rather than the ego, we can see ourselves as magnificent beings with a physical body that we must value and for which we are responsible. The fact that we're secure in our own identity allows us, without jealousy or envy, to also have joy in the success and empowerment of others.

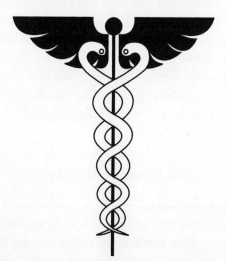

Figure 6: The ancient representation of the kundalini is the caduceus. It depicts two snakes coiling around a central staff meeting at the highest point before giving way to a pair of outstretched wings. It's the universal emblem of healing and medicine.

Spiritual Awakening

Over the centuries, mystics have described the immense power of the root chakra by likening it to a snake, the kundalini, which lies coiled, asleep within the pelvis. It waits to be awakened only when spiritual development is sufficiently advanced to allow us to cope with its power.

When the kundalini begins to rise, its energy can travel quite rapidly within the central energy channel up the whole length of the spine, passing through every other chakra on its way. It emerges at the level of the seventh chakra, having cleared and revitalized the whole system, opening the way to spiritual freedom.

The crown center and all those in between can be open and functioning without the raising of the kundalini having occurred. However, in practical terms, a sign that the first chakra is open and the kundalini has risen is that the person has true charisma, not to be confused with charm. It's a quality which encompasses a strong sense of self, with good esteem and self-worth, but without conceit or arrogance. Charismatic individuals attract others with their power and appeal, while healing energy flows from and around them. Usually the charismatic is not only working from a powerful base, but has balance in the other chakras too and is blessed with humility since the power is spiritual and does not come from the ego.

Sexual Pleasure

Although it's the second chakra (the sacral) that's associated with our sexuality, the first is the one that governs the basic instinct of sex.

If the root chakra is closed, we're robbed of a totally different quality of sexual pleasure that's only available when the powers of the first and second chakras combine. True orgasm which, unlike mere ejaculation, involves and encompasses the whole being, can only occur when the root chakra gives us the stability to let go with complete abandon. For that, we need an open base chakra to know that we can soar to the heavens in ecstasy but remain whole and safe to return here when we're ready.

As the fountain of energy flows upwards, each chakra lends its individual power to the sexual experience. The sexuality of each partner is awakened at the second chakra; the power of the union is felt at the third. The heart chakra lends love, the throat offers communication. There is vision at the brow chakra and as the energy reaches each partner's crown there's a flood of spiritual energy that produces a symphony of sensations. This gives an experience far beyond any previous understanding of sexual pleasure and beyond mere physical

---

RAISING THE KUNDALINI

Much has been written about the dangers of attempting to raise the kundalini prematurely and, although there's no need to be nervous about the work as it is prescribed here, there is a need to respect the extraordinary power of this base center. Premature raising of the kundalini has accounted for some episodes of disturbed behavior which are often mistaken for psychosis. Admittedly, the shock of a rapid and sometimes explosive opening of all the chakras without the right support and expertise can result in distressing behavior. If the spiritual nature of the experience is missed (and the chances of this are greatly increased when a patient is strongly medicated), then healing, recovery and further development can be obstructed or delayed.

This situation should not be confused with other psychiatric illnesses. I'm not implying that all people suffering from psychotic experience are really having a kundalini awakening or other spiritual emergency, but the possibility is worth investigating.

Some powerful healing and grounding usually helps in these situations, but prescribed medication and the advice of medical practitioners should not be ignored or rejected.

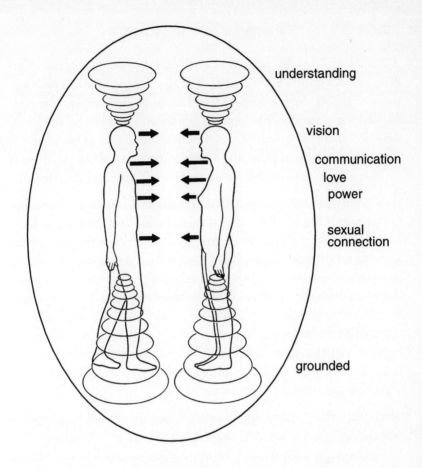

understanding

vision

communication
love
power

sexual
connection

grounded

Figure 7: Orgasm—both remain grounded but open to each other in sexual connection, with power and will, mutual loving, good communication and vision of their union. There is a spiritual experience with great awareness and understanding, and the auras blend.

experience. It raises the sexual act to the heights of spiritual experience and orgasm to a unique event that, with practice, can be prolonged until every bit of healing is exacted from it.

Without the first chakra in optimum health, this all-embracing emotional, mental, physical and spiritual release cannot take place. That can leave a feeling of disappointment and frustration with sexual intimacy since its depths can never be plumbed, nor its heights reached.

Damage to the Root Chakra

All of the chakras are present at birth in a rudimentary form. However, the root chakra is the first to undergo change, its major development occurring during the first few months of life. Very early trauma will therefore usually cause some dysfunction at the level of our primitive will to survive. Our sense of individuality and personal worth may be affected to the point that there's ambivalence about life, in some cases leading to such self-loathing that there's active suicidal intent.

Less florid dysfunction at this chakra can manifest itself as a tendency to opt out of life in other ways—to dissociate and drift away, emotionally and psychologically absenting ourselves from the present and seeming to drift out of the body altogether. I remember one young woman who would spend much of her sessions with me staring into the space between us or focusing somewhere behind my shoulder. She floated outside herself, in a place totally inaccessible to me. She'd suffered some brutal treatment very early in her life and when she became well enough to talk about it, she recounted how she used to float out and leave her body during that time so as to simply watch what was happening but no longer feel it.

Sometimes this "absenting" happens when people are in a particularly stressful situation. Although it can be due to difficulties at the brow chakra, if it's a regular feature, and especially if it's associated with a history of early trauma, it's much more likely to be a problem of the root chakra. This particular woman managed to confront the painful issues she needed to heal by learning to stay in her body. To do this, she repeatedly grounded herself using the exercises at the end of this chapter.

If you experience root chakra problems, you may also encounter existential crises, accompanied by a rumbling disquiet and a questioning of the value of life and creation in general. This leads to cynicism and an inability to appreciate the wonder of the universe on any level. Such undervaluing of the planet and the environment eventually results in internal anarchy with a breakdown of generally accepted social values and norms. This can spread beyond the individual to become a problem of the local subculture and eventually of the planet itself.

Over the last century, the whole planet has been experiencing a root chakra problem which is now being worked through with a return to more wholesome and earthy values. The emergence of a wealth of "green" food stores and spiritual workshops (and your purchase of this book) attests to that movement.

Children learn by example from their parents and other authority figures such as school teachers. If there's a disregard for social values, or if those demonstrated are distorted or pernicious, then the next generation is doubly damaged by such exposure. For example, the child who witnesses and therefore learns racism is not only learning a negative way of responding to his or her environment, but also is suffering the loss of the enriching influence of other cultures and the experience integration brings.

The overall outcome is either a lack of development or the active distortion of the child's base chakra, or both. Communities where respect for the planet has been lost perpetuate transgenerational damage to the root chakra. Children in these circumstances develop little sense of self and are usually unable to esteem themselves or others, though they may compensate for this by the development of a kind of arrogance which at least allows the growing ego to function in what is perceived as a hostile world. Another child, even in a materially deprived environment, who is taught to appreciate what there is, however little that may be, will be well grounded with a strong root chakra and a strong sense of self-worth. He will have a desire to be alive, to achieve and to fulfill his potential with a will to nurture himself and be open to nurturing others.

Painful, deprived (not necessarily materially) and suffering parents who are trying to cope within painful, deprived and suffering communities are often unable to give their children the kind of positive modeling and nurturing they need. There are parents who are very affluent but who are still deprived in many ways. They struggle with their own damage and a suffering "inner child," while valiantly

trying to be parents. Sometimes the very fact of being highly materially privileged prompts a lifestyle that prevents parents from having
much contact time with their children, so the child develops little
sense of who she is except in terms of title and status.

I've seen many young (and older) people from privileged backgrounds
who have little sense of grounding. They've often had so much that
they have little sense of the value of anything and are restless and lost.
Their lack of need has often led them to be wasteful of the resources
they have, internal as well as material, and thus they have no real
sense of worth. Nonetheless, they may sometimes behave in a superior, prima donna fashion. Helping them get grounded by working on
the root chakra is the first task. Often they begin to blossom very
quickly as they start to feel real for the first time and are able to see
that they have resources (internal and external) that are valuable to
themselves and others when used for the higher good of all.

Frequently, it's society's inability to nurture, protect and support both
our children and their parents in a positive environment that results
in self-perpetuating dysfunction. Sadly, negativity is around us constantly, and robs many of the anticipation of prosperity, both material
and spiritual, even before they start. A society that's constantly preach-
ing that there'll be no work for those who drop out of school no matter how well they do denies them hope and the possibility of developing entrepreneurial skills that are latent and just need a little
encouragement.

As a parent, please be compassionate with yourself as well as with
your children and your own parents. Try not to chastise yourself or
hold guilt for anything you may have done while parenting—though
as a parent myself, I know how painful it can be.

I truly believe that we have all been doing the best we could in the
light of our understanding, the information we have and our own
physical, mental and emotional state. Our parents were doing the
same, as were their parents before them. The old cliche that we are all
victims of victims is very true. With hindsight, and now coming from
a different standpoint emotionally, mentally and spiritually, I for one
would have done things differently. But I know I did my best as a par-

ent and I need to forgive myself and ask my children for their forgiveness for what I got wrong, which was a considerable amount.

If we're to be our own loving parent, to be open to our growth, to be fully alive, happy, and to have good relationships both with ourselves and with others, then there's no substitute for the work that needs to be done at this chakra. So, to become the best you can be, the work has to begin here, and the following exercises and meditations will help.

How to Get the Best from the Exercises

Each of the following exercises will improve the performance of your root chakra and promote its cleansing and good functioning. The exercises can be repeated as often as you like and in any order you choose. Even when you progress to higher chakras, these exercises can still be valuable and can be repeated at any time. However, you should always take yourself to your safe place and make yourself comfortable to work. Take your notebook with you, as you'll need this for both the exercises and the meditations. Light a candle if you wish and take as long as you need.

If you have a crystal, keep it close by. A clear quartz would be fine, though stones especially good for work with your root chakra are smoky quartz, garnet or bloodstone. All three of these are good for your sexual energy, and promote balance. The bloodstone, as its name suggests, also has healing properties for the blood and will help keep you centered while you work. The smoky quartz will help you settle down to meditate while also being helpful for ridding you of negativity and skepticism. Garnet is a lovely and inexpensive stone that is wonderful for balancing your libido with the emotional and spiritual components of sex. It has effects on the higher chakras (as do the other crystals) and enhances love, compassion and imagination. If you have a ring or other piece of jewelry with a ruby in it, that would be good to wear as long as you clean it (see earlier instructions for keeping your crystals clean). Ruby is a strong stone that can increase harmony and balance while being full of power and passion—just like the root chakra itself.

If you want to vaporize some oil or burn incense, lavender, sandal-wood, cedar or patchouli would be appropriate. If you have access to an aromatherapist, I'm sure she will mix a blend that's right for you. As with all the chakras, while you're doing the work on a particular area you can use the oils in several ways to keep your atmosphere balanced while hopefully not upsetting anyone else in your environment. Scented candles, oil vaporizers and having a soak in the bath with a few drops of the appropriate oil will be very healing for you, but please check with fellow residents that they don't mind having your fragrance in their space. Perfumes know no boundaries and I have known people who are irritated by the presence of "New Age smells."

Exercise 1

Think of five things you would like to do. They may be things you used to enjoy—for example spending a day at the beach, having an evening just by yourself curled up with a book, having a massage—or something totally new. Then make a realistic date with yourself to do them. Mark it in your diary. Some things you may be able to begin right away, others may take some preparation, but there's always a first step that can begin almost immediately. For example if you decide to take a holiday, the first step may be to get some travel brochures or book time off work. If you want to start a course of massage or aromatherapy, then start to look for a good therapist.

Try to include some activity that involves contact with the earth—taking a walk in the forest, walking on the beach in bare feet, collecting shells, wild flowers, pine cones or pretty leaves. Maybe you could make a collage with them when you come home or arrange them in your safe place on an altar.

The appointments you make with yourself are as important as the appointments you make with anyone else. So try to respect them and keep them as you would with anyone else. If for some reason you do have to break a commitment to yourself, reschedule as soon as possible and carry through your promise to this very important new person in your life—yourself.

Exercise 2

Treat yourself to something as a reward for taking the first step on the journey to self-healing. Please don't think you have to buy a whole host of supplies. Maybe some simple candles (night-lights will do) and the oil/incense or a single crystal for this particular chakra is enough. An oil vaporizer is useful, but a saucer with a few drops of oil and some boiling water will do. Please be careful with the hot water and lighted candles, and never leave them unattended. Whatever you purchase, make a relationship with it. Touch it, feel it, enjoy it, develop a light excited feeling about having it. Really appreciate it—realizing its value will help you appreciate your own.

Exercise 3

Write in your journal anything that comes to mind about your base chakra. Try to develop the technique of writing without taking your hand off the page to think, rewrite or correct anything. Just let your hand continue to write, even if you're stuck and feel silly anyway. Eventually, your logical left brain will empty and allow your more creative right brain to communicate. You might be amazed at what happens.

A common problem here is getting started. If that's so, I suggest you begin by writing: "This is really silly. I don't know why Brenda asked me to do it and I just feel foolish. I really don't have anything to write about. What do I know about my root chakra? But I remember that when I was a little girl/boy . . ." Then you're off. If you get stuck, just keep writing: "Now I'm stuck. I don't have anything else to say. This is really a pain and I don't really want to do it. It's a waste of time anyway. Oh, I do remember . . ." And you're off again.

No one's going to read this but you, so you can say whatever you want. What will happen is that you'll suddenly start to talk from your creative self without the inhibition of your logical brain. We'll use this technique again and again so allow yourself fifteen or twenty minutes, with the agreement with yourself that you won't take your hand off the page unless there's a fire!

Grounding Exercises

Whatever work we are doing, it's essential to remember that we are spiritual beings in human form and that we need to remain rooted to the earth.

So many people who embark on spiritual work forget this and become so cut off from their lower chakras that they have an airy-fairy feeling around them that not only robs them of the security of their root chakra, leaving them open and vulnerable, but also does untold harm to the whole healing and complementary medicine movement. Beware those who seem to be floating around on some higher plane. Those who are really in touch spiritually are very human and ordinary, albeit in an extraordinary way. Being grounded will eventually become second nature, but, just like protection, it's important to do it properly and not cut corners. Grounding is something we need to do at the end of every exercise, every meditation and at any time when we feel a little lost or that things are a bit unreal. It's also very comforting and makes us feel strong since it taps into the power of the earth and holds us steady and sturdy like a huge tree.

METHOD 1

Sit or stand with your back erect if you can, with your feet flat on the ground and a little apart so that you're well balanced.

If you're standing, let your whole weight sit in your pelvis and be distributed equally down your legs with your knees just slightly bent. You may like to close your eyes.

Take a few deep breaths and relax as much as you can. With a single thought send a beautiful golden root from the sole of each foot deep down into the earth. Send another from the tip of your spine so that you are now sitting on a tripod of golden roots. Just as a lightning rod grounds electrical energy, if there's anything you don't need, allow it to discharge now into the earth. Just let it go. The earth can handle anything, neutralize and recycle it.

Now with each breath, draw up the wonderful energy of the earth. Feel it hold you and nourish you as it comes up through those roots and into your body. See it begin to fill you with wonderful golden light. Strong, earthy, robust energy.

Feel held by the earth. Like a wonderful strong tree, know that you too are strong and that you're fine. Stay as long as you like.

When you're ready, gently withdraw the roots, but know that you remain in constant, intimate contact with the earth through the soles of your feet and your root chakra, which should remain open.

METHOD 2

I love to do this barefoot on the earth. Stand erect if you can, with your feet slightly apart and flat on the ground. Send down a root from the sole of each foot and from your root chakra. With a single thought, discharge anything into the earth that you no longer need.

Now, draw up the golden energy of the earth through all three roots. Feel the wonderful sturdy energy fill you. Draw it up to the level of your heart so that it fills and surrounds your heart like a flaming golden ball. Feel how wonderful that is. Breathe into it and enjoy it.

Now put your hands up to the sky and draw the energy of the sun and the sky through the palms of your hands and the top of your head. Let this wonderful silver energy fill you, streaming in and down to your heart where it mingles with the energy of the earth.

Silently or aloud give thanks for all the good there ever was, for all the good there is and for all the good that's to come. Feel the strength from both earth and sky flow into you and hold you, mingling the earthly and the spiritual, the perfect marriage of your human self with your eternal soul. Feel with wonder the current of energy flow through you. Enjoy it. Feel the strength. Feel the power. Feel refreshed and renewed. Know that you are a powerful being, your physical self enriched by the spiritual and your spiritual self humble in its human form. Feel the magic of that amazing union. Feel whole, be aware of your immense potential. Feel energized.

When you are ready, bring down your arms and cup your hands around your heart. Say whatever you need to say in thanks. Holding on to the wonderful energy of both earth and sky, withdraw the roots from the earth, but know that you always remain in intimate contact with it through your open root chakra.

The Meditations

It's essential to do the meditations in the order in which they're given to obtain maximum benefit. You can repeat them as often as you wish, and in the future you may want to do only the second meditation. That's fine. Before you start, make sure you read the following section on forgiveness.

> Forgiveness is in three stages. Don't worry if you're not ready to proceed through all of them right now. With this and every chakra, you can come back and repeat the meditations whenever you want to and it may take some time before you feel you can do it all. That's fine. Don't push yourself. It may be that you have to proceed further and understand more before you feel you can forgive fully. We'll be coming back to forgiveness when we get to the heart chakra. But for now, here are those stages.

> *Stage 1*—If I do something to hurt you and I say I'm sorry you can forgive me for what I did.

> *Stage 2*—You can come to realize that whatever I did, I did because of my own process and what was going on in my life at the time. My anger or irritability or the way I treated you was not really about you but about the difficulties I was having. You can understand and forgive me with compassion.

> *Stage 3*—You can rise to the highest spiritual perspective and realize that you set various lessons for yourself in this lifetime and so you needed someone to help you learn those lessons. For example, if I needed to learn about betrayal, then I needed someone to betray me. Now, from this place, you can forgive me with love, compassion, understanding and gratitude.

Meditation 1

Go to your safe place and take the phone off the hook. Give yourself about forty-five minutes without disturbance to complete this meditation. Be as comfortable as you can with your spine as erect as possible, using whatever support you need, and your feet firmly on the floor. If you are disabled or, for some reason, unable to meditate sitting upright, it's possible to do so lying down. Some people favor the classic cross-legged yoga position.

Now . . . take a deep breath and hold the air for a moment to extract the goodness from it. Enjoy, and when you breathe out let any impurities flow out in your breath. Take another deep breath and this time, as you breathe out, allow your body to relax: let your shoulders fall, let your chair take your weight, let anything negative flow out through your root chakra and through the soles of your feet. Relax. Repeat this, taking your time. Let yourself breathe in the goodness of the air, the energy that you've created in your safe place with your crystals and oil. Then when you breathe out, let a wave of relaxation pass through you as you let go of anything you no longer need. Now, take your focus back and back and back in time. You're going back to the point of your conception. Back to the moment when one cell from your mother and one cell from your father joined and your physical being was created.

Back to the time when you were warm and safe in your mother's womb. And now, I want you to wrap the time, events and people of that time and up to the age of about five in a parcel that you're going to heal. You don't have to remember the details unless you want to.

Wrap your child self of that time securely in love, holding gently, holding firmly, holding with healing love and light.

And now, with your child self still held gently but securely, wrapped in love and light in your heart, be gentle with yourself. Take your time. If, at any time, you feel you're not ready to proceed, simply stop. Return using your grounding exercise (see page 78) and gently bring your focus back to the room. You do not have to do the whole process today. You can return to it when you're ready.

If you are ready to proceed . . .

Send out a beam of light to the time, the places, the events, the people of those first five years from conception. A beam of bright, white light to flow into, around, over and through the people, the events, the time and particularly yourself. Now, let the past be healed and release yourself from it. Let it be healed. Let it go. Whatever happened then is over. It's complete. You can choose to let it go. You've survived it. Be free of it. Let it be healed.

Let the light spread over all the time and events from your conception till you were five. Let it spread out to envelop everything and every person of that time. Release it. Let it go, bathed in light, be free.

And now, if you can, raise yourself to a higher spiritual level and see that the people who may have hurt you then were living out their own pain and their own process. They behaved as they did because of their own difficulties. Send out a beam of light and forgive them. Forgive them and let them go, so that you no longer need to hold on to anything of that time that will stop you from moving on and fulfilling your potential. Send them forgiveness. Send them light. Free them. Free yourself. Let them go, let them go in light.

Now, if you can, raise yourself to an even higher spiritual level and see that without the people, the events, the pain of that time, you could not have learned all that you needed to know. All that you had set yourself to learn. See that the people who were part of your process were essential to your total life journey. And from this highest spiritual perspective, send them love, send them gratitude, and set them free of their burden of guilt.

Feel cleansed and enjoy the healing. Allow the sense of freedom to percolate through you as you're free for the first time. Allow a beam of light to come into the top of your head and gently spread through you as you enjoy your inner peace. Take your time . . . enjoy.

When you're ready, be aware that your child self is secure in your heart where you can visit as often as you wish. Now you're going to prepare to come back to the room. Bring your focus gently up through your body. Feel your fingers and toes. Be aware of your physical presence. Let your focus now be behind your eyes as you are more and more aware of your surroundings. Put your arms around your physical body and, gently, when you're ready, open your eyes.

Have a drink of water and record whatever you wish in your journal. Then take a rest before you do the final root chakra meditation.

Meditation 2

Wearing some comfortable clothes and, choosing a time when you won't be disturbed, go to your safe place. Take the phone off the hook. Have a comfortable chair to sit on so that your feet touch the floor and your back can be upright, supported if necessary. If you're more comfortable sitting on the floor, then do so, but with your back upright. Close your eyes and for a moment focus on your breathing.

Take a deep breath in and hold it for just a few seconds to allow your lungs to extract the goodness from the air before you breathe out. Breathe out all the way and, as you do so, let any tension or anxiety flow out with your breath. This time, take a deep breath and feel yourself taking in the healing from the air, then allow yourself to breathe all the way out, and as you do so, let your body relax, your shoulders fall, let your chair take your weight and allow anything negative to simply flow out through the soles of your feet. Relax.

Take another deep breath and this time, as you breathe out, let out a long sigh and visualize any impurities flowing out of your body in your breath. Relax.

Now gently take your focus down through the center of your body until it rests in your pelvis. Imagine your pelvis like a bowl, the bottom of which is sitting at your perineum, that area between your anus and your vagina or scrotum. This is the site of your root chakra. Here at the bottom of the beautiful bowl that is your pelvis there is a wonderful red light, like a deep crimson setting sun. Feel the warmth of this light in your pelvis. Feel the sensation of the energy there. See if you can perceive any movement, any change in the color as you focus on it. Send some loving feelings to this area if you can and feel the whole area respond with warmth. Focus for as long as you wish on this beautiful red swirling, bright, shining, sparkling light. If you perceive any other color here, just with a breath, allow it to change to red. If you cannot see a color at all, don't worry. Sometimes the visualization takes practice. It will come.

Allow this red light to spread gently down both of your legs, filling your thighs and revitalizing your muscles, tendons, nerves—every cell and every atom of every cell being filled with the light. Let it continue to spread down through your legs, pushing ahead of it anything you don't need in this area—any tension, stiffness, any blocks. Just breathe away any resistance until you can allow a free flow of this beautiful energy—warming, cleansing and healing—filling your legs now . . . cleansing . . . healing . . . energizing. Let it now enter into your feet, again entering every cell, every atom. When you feel as though your whole legs and feet are filled with the light, let it flow out through the soles of your feet and down into the earth where it forms deep roots anchoring you to the wonderful earth energy, holding you secure and solid in the mother earth. At the same time, send a root down directly from your base chakra. Down, down into the earth so that you're now supported and rooted in three areas, holding you secure and strong. Feel a warm sense of security, of belonging, of knowing you are part of this planet, this universe. Feel the warmth, security and comfort of belonging here in your chosen place.

Stay for as long as you wish holding this connection with the earth, feeling secure, feeling held by the earth. Feel your roots deep down within the body of the living earth. Like a strong tree, you are rooted and steady. You belong.

Now it's time to allow the earth to nurture you. With a breath, draw up the healing energy of the earth through the roots you've sunk deep into it. See this as golden energy, healing energy, vital energy, energy of everything good there ever was, now being given freely to you—to heal you, to make you strong, to make you well. Let this energy move up through your legs, through your thighs and into the power center upon which you are sitting—the root chakra. See the golden energy of the earth mingle with the crimson energy of this beautiful spinning chakra—the healing energy of the earth mixing with your own energy. Feel the healing as the fresh power comes in to bathe you and make you whole. See the petals of the chakra open even further as you welcome the powerful energy of the earth and allow the healing to occur. Feel yourself rooted to the planet and feel a sense of your own power as a living part of the universe being fed by the mother earth.

Savor the feeling of this whole area being energized with beautiful crimson light as the energy of the planet continues to flow in.

Now, gather up that energy and, with a breath, allow it to gently move up through your body, healing as it goes. Gently up through every organ, filling you with that same sense of wholeness and belonging. All of you now being filled with the energy of the earth and becoming stronger. Feel yourself fully present in this moment, in your body. Let the energy continue to rise gently until eventually it sprays out through the top of your head and, like a fountain, falls gently around you, shimmering through your aura and falling back down to the earth. As you breathe, allow the energy to flow as you sit now in this living fountain of light, energizing and strengthening you from within and energizing your aura as it falls again back to the earth. As you breathe, feel your self as part of this living fountain. You may find that the light has taken on a different color. As it rises it may have become golden, or pink, or white. Allow yourself to be showered in it as the flow continues, healing and cleansing you as you remain rooted to the earth.

Stay for as long as you wish. Enjoy the feeling. Stay rooted and grounded. Centered in your physical body but enjoying the movement, the flow, the never-ending motion of the energy as it passes through you. Each time you breathe, be aware of your part in the constant motion, the constant cycle of the universe—energy flowing in, up through you and cascading down around you, back to the earth, joining you to the earth. Know that in this moment, you have all you need and more. In this moment, you are home with the earth where you belong.

Gradually, when you're ready, allow the flow to slow down and stop while still holding the feelings of security and belonging. You are still rooted to the earth. Now you're going to gently withdraw those roots but remain in intimate contact with the earth. With a thought and a breath and giving thanks to the earth for its healing energy, allow the roots to withdraw, gently, slowly, bringing with them the last bit of energy they can carry. Allow the soles of your feet to close as the energy now continues to withdraw. Draw it up your legs and into your pelvis, the crimson light localizing again deep in your pelvis where it resides. But know that you will continue to allow the nurturing of your legs and feet and of all your body with the strong earthy energy

---

ADDICTION

The reasons for starting to use addictive substances and the reasons for continuing to do so differ. There's usually some early trauma leading to a poor sense of self-worth and lack of inner security that results from distortion at the root chakra. The need to escape reality prompts a search for some way of being absent, at least for a while, in a vain hope that the problem will go away. Of course, the underlying problems of poor self-esteem, feelings of loss, abandonment and lack of belonging are only exacerbated as the guilt and shame add to a spiraling sense of defeat.

The addictive substance then has a life of its own. There's now intoxication, excessive consumption and dependence to add to the original problems and it's these that make it even more difficult to stop. The ultimate outcome is an increase in the sense of separation, isolation and loss, often accompanied by a disregard for the home and surroundings and a drifting down the social scale as any residual sense of grounding or belonging is eroded.

There's also the new damage to brain cells to add to the problem and a very dangerous situation develops as ambivalence about being alive gives way to a desire to be dead. Work at the root chakra can often arrest the cycle long enough for the chemical effects of the addictive substance to subside so that the real work can begin.

of your base. You are now fully within your physical body. Allow yourself to affirm your intention to remain grounded and whole.

Silently say these affirmations (see Glossary, page 228 and Chapter 8, page 159 for a fuller explanation):

> I am a beloved child of the universe and I deserve love, peace and security.
>
> I open myself to receive the abundance of the universe.
>
> I am open to receive and accept love.
>
> I am open to receive and be nurtured by the powerful energy of the earth.
>
> I am a physical being and value my physical presence.
>
> I resolve to take care of my body and accept it as it is today.
>
> I value it as the physical temple in which I live and I will aim to provide for its needs in terms of food, rest, stimulation and general nurturing.

Gently add any affirmation you wish.

When you feel you're ready, give thanks in whatever way you choose. Then, gently start your return to the room. Be aware of your physical body. Move your fingers and toes and gently stretch. When you're ready, feeling your feet firmly on the ground, open your eyes. Stay where you are for a little while until you feel ready to move. Be gentle with yourself.

Make yourself a warm drink or have some water and write in your journal anything you wish to record.

When you feel ready to do so, put your phone back on the hook.

FIVE

The Sacral Chakra: Sexual Healing

∽

The bride comes from the heart of dawn,
And the bridegroom from the sunset.
There is a wedding in the valley.
A day too vast for recording.

—*Kahlil Gibran*

As the root chakra is essentially about survival, stability and grounding, the sacral is about movement, flexibility and flow. The earthy energy of the root gives us a good base to stand on, from which we can start to reach out into the world. We've developed a relationship with ourselves and now we can start to look outward and toward having relationships with others: the fountain of energy we began to use in the meditation of the last chapter is rising and gaining force.

The work we've already done has helped us gain a healthy sense of self. We now have enough internal stability, strength and security to begin to cope with relationships. We can begin to expand and grow and move beyond ourselves, flowing toward others and starting to commune with them. Whereas our focus previously was only on our inner self, now we can start to look outward at our relationship with the world, embracing it on a personal level with friends and lovers, in family, in our social life and, in a broader sense, within a global community.

Though the basic instincts of the base chakra ensured sex and the survival of the species, it's here at the sacral that we begin to be able to feel sexual intimacy. We begin our personal transformation as we stimulate our creativity for the first time. Although creativity is enhanced at the throat chakra, its release here ensures that we'll be able to make the most of the next chakra, the solar plexus, and achieve our potential.

Here the accent is on flow. Try to keep your mind on that concept and you'll feel the gentle push of energy rising up through you. This is the first flow of inspiration as the higher centers are also stimulated into action.

The color of this chakra is bright orange. It's located about three inches below the navel and emits shining translucent, iridescent light in all directions. Its glow fills the pelvis, bathing the sexual organs, enlivening our desire and capacity for pleasure. Its element is water and though it's associated with the reproductive system, especially in women (the penis is root chakra property!), it also energizes and balances those organs associated with the movement of fluid, namely the renal system (kidneys, ureters and bladder), the lymphatics, and to some extent blood circulation. Its function is to keep everything gently moving, ebbing and flowing.

Touching You, Touching Me

The sacral is also the center for nurturing and tenderness. It prompts us to take care of ourselves and to care for others, and to enjoy both the giving and receiving of sensual (not necessarily sexual) pleasure.

The need for touch and nurturing is as basic as the need for food and water. Children who are deprived of adequate touch fail to thrive as well as those who may have considerably less materially. A classic experiment some years ago showed that baby monkeys given a wire "mother" that dispensed milk refused to play and failed to develop well, even though they were adequately fed. Those given the same conditions, except that a piece of fur covered the wire "mother," snuggled and climbed and generally thrived happily.

Ideally our mothers model nurturing as they gently care for us and we learn to do the same to others. As the woman caresses her child, the baby learns to touch and explore. As we grow, touch becomes a major form of communication, whether as parents cuddling our own children, strangers meeting with a handshake, friends giving affection or comfort or as lovers giving sexual pleasure. Without adequate touch, we're isolated and cold, cut off from the warmth and joy of another human being's skin in contact with ours. Making an effort to touch someone—even just brushing the hand of the cashier at the supermarket checkout as she gives you your change—will make a subtle difference to your day. However, do make touch appropriate and be sure you have permission before rushing in to hug someone.

Exploring Sexuality

With a healthy sacral chakra, we begin to enjoy touching as well as being touched, giving as well as receiving. In the sexual sphere, we move from demanding what we want to enjoying giving as part of the transaction: from the merely biological, functional aspect of sex, with its focus on procreation (the function of the root chakra), to using sexual intimacy as a form of communication, mutual comfort and nurturing.

The focus shifts from "me" to "us," and the desire to please as well as to have becomes a major part of the equation. Here we refine sex and lust to desire and love. There now develops a sense of holding the beloved in love. For most couples this is a major part of healthy, long-term bonding. Marvin Gaye's song "Sexual Healing" sums up this aspect of the sacral chakra.

Men and women experience sexual intimacy and desire quite differently. Intimacy of any kind is generally a much deeper and more rapidly developing phenomenon for women. Note the marked difference in the level of warmth and intimacy between female friends to that shared by most men. Women who enjoy a sexually intimate relationship with another woman report a much deeper, more spiritual relationship than they've experienced with a man.

Most women tend to tap into a deep sense of spirituality associated with their sexuality, whereas men are much more governed by their physical equipment. Remember again that the penis is governed by the root chakra, which deals with basic instincts. The female genitalia, however, are in the sacral area. Since women's cyclical flow mirrors other natural phenomena, such as the moon and the tides, they are naturally more bound to the elements and spirituality.

Men may take longer to develop a sense of intimacy and commitment, but those who are open at this chakra are capable of enduring dedication, which includes the desire to protect and provide for their partner with a deep and spiritual passion.

When two people who are spiritually open at the sacral chakra come together, there's often an accompanying sense of having known each other forever, of being meant to be together. This holds true in any combination of the sexes. We'll be looking at this phenomenon of karmic connectedness when we discuss relationships in greater detail in Chapter 7.

Reaching an Internal Balance

Our sexuality allows for the coming together of the masculine and the feminine, but this isn't only an external phenomenon. The coming together of the masculine and the feminine also takes place within each of us as we develop spiritually, whether or not we have a partner.

The masculine element—the part of us that deals with action, logic, organization, ambition and drive (and a host of other things)—is governed by the left brain. The feminine, right-brain functions include verbal skills, creativity, music, art and other less structured gifts. Development of the sacral chakra moves us toward a state of internal balance between our masculine (action) and feminine (nurturing) principles. Let's look at this in a little more detail.

Within the healthy, mature, heterosexual man, the masculine principle will generally be to the fore, though when appropriate, he'll be comfortable and willing to accept and display the softer more feminine aspects of his character. Young men often have difficulty accepting their feminine element and may compensate by displaying a macho image. The same man twenty years later behaves very differently as he's now more balanced and much more at ease with his feminine aspect.

In the healthy, mature, heterosexual woman, the feminine principle is well supported by the masculine within her so that she can be soft, warm and loving, but still be organized, with ambition and drive. In her earlier days, she may have been more flighty before she developed the balance with her inner masculine principle. Remember the concept of flow. It's the fluidity of the healthy sacral chakra that facilitates constant change and movement between the masculine and feminine principles, flexibility being the hallmark of the healthy adult.

Let me give you an example. I may be in my usual working state with my feminine aspect to the fore. I'm loving, being as creative as I can while searching for solutions and embracing whoever I'm working with in healing energy. But my masculine element is very much in support, helping me organize my thoughts and express them in an easily understandable form. Should there suddenly be a threat from any area—let's say there's a fire—my masculine principle would spring to the fore and take action. It would help me organize, make plans, command as necessary and be as aggressive as the situation demands in order to save the people in my care and to ensure that the building is evacuated as quickly and efficiently as possible.

During this process, my whole demeanor would be different—my voice in both its tone and its delivery, my movements, my thinking, my approach—and though I would exhibit great care and the feminine Brenda would still be there, it is my masculine principle that would protect and lead the way until the crisis was resolved. There may be other crises in which having the feminine element to the fore is much more appropriate. In a volatile, aggressive situation, the power of the gentle, loving feminine is much better at defusing the situation effectively. This phenomenon is so well recognized that women are often employed in situations where there's a potential for violence, such as in male prisons and in crisis intervention teams. The presence of women has been shown to minimize violent incidents. Yet these women need to be well balanced, with their feminine principle to the fore but very closely supported by the masculine principle that remains vigilant, ready to protect and to act if a change of tactic is required.

In cases where life events and trauma have resulted in dysfunction at this chakra, or if there's a failure to gain maturity, a flexible internal balance between the masculine and feminine is impossible. The result is rigidity, not only within ourselves but also in our relationships with others.

Imbalance internally results in imbalance in relationships. We've all seen couples where the woman in the relationship is carrying most of the masculine element (Have you ever said, "She wears the pants in that household"?) and the man is carrying more of the feminine. The result is that the man appears "henpecked" and the woman never has her needs fulfilled.

There are relationships too in which both partners carry a lot of masculine. In this situation, there's constant butting of heads and aggression from both sides, with neither willing to nurture the other and neither having their needs met. Where there seems to be very little masculine in evidence from either partner, even if they mean to care for each other, the whole relationship lacks direction or drive, and there's chaos. What's lost in all of these relationships is not only balance but flexibility.

Conversely, in a healthy couple, each is secure within their sexuality, there's flow and movement internally and therefore they can switch roles regularly. Let's say the man has an accident. If necessary, the woman can take over the masculine functions within the relationship at a moment's notice. She'll immediately slip into organizing everything that needs to be done (many women will see this as their usual function in any case). She'll protect him, aggressively if necessary, she'll organize and direct. Similarly, the balanced male can switch into a gentler, more nurturing role. However, the healthy, well-balanced couple won't wait for a crisis, and they will also alternate in sex.

Please remember, I'm talking about internal masculine and feminine principles here and not about men and women or male versus female roles—I don't want to start a riot! So, when the sacral chakra is functioning well, the healthy adult has enough internal balance of masculine and feminine to achieve a self-confident balance in their relationships with others. There can be a coming together and sharing on all levels and with all functions. Both partners can share the caring, the budgeting, the working, the organizing, the planning, the housework, etc., as they flow within themselves as individuals and within the bounds of their relationship. Two separate people who nevertheless are a couple working as a team.

Usually we choose a partner who balances our own sexuality. So a man with a very strong masculine principle may look for a woman who's very feminine whom he can look after and dominate and who doesn't challenge him. The woman in this relationship will be well partnered by such a man since she has little sense of her own masculine principle and will be looking for a father-type figure to take care of her. On the other hand, a man with a poorly developed masculine principle may look for a strong, dominant female who'll take charge and relieve him of much that is expected of him as a man, so that he feels less challenged within himself. The woman in this partnership is looking for someone who'll allow her masculine element plenty of room.

Though these relationships may appear to give each partner balance overall, imagine what happens when either of them starts to grow spiritually and "get well." The more the internal balance of one improves, the more unstable the relationship can become. The partner is threatened and often makes counter-moves to keep his or her loved one "sick" so that the status quo is preserved. Ideally, one partner getting well prompts the other to do so too (see Chapter 7 for more on loving relationships).

Taken to its logical conclusion, we could have someone who's so well balanced within that she or he has no need to look externally for an opposite partner. This is a highly evolved person who is self-sufficient, fluid, flexible and has good, strong energy from the sacral chakra that helps balance all the chakras above and the root chakra below. They may still choose to fall in love and be with someone, but there's less need to search for an opposite mate, for the opposite is contained within themselves.

Their relationships succeed on the basis of wanting rather than needing another. Some may feel threatened at the prospect of not being needed, but it's a much greater statement of love to be where we are because we want to be rather than because we need to be. In healthy, loving relationships, co-dependent need that leaves us feeling incomplete unless we're intimately involved with another is replaced by choice and desire.

And what of gay couples? In the stable couple, the masculine and feminine are still generally balanced overall and the same principles apply. It may be that one partner carries more of the feminine and chooses a partner who complements this by carrying more of the masculine, or vice versa. In some couples, each person has achieved that internal balance whereby they're beyond the need for further balancing from outside themselves.

Falling in Love

We'll be dealing with falling in love and the state of loving in further detail in Chapter 7 but, since the sacral is so intimately involved, it needs to be mentioned here.

When two people find each other sexually attractive and fall in love, the sacral center opens, and with it the heart chakra, which deals with human loving. The throat chakra, which governs ideas and communication, also opens quite suddenly and it is this connection between the throat and the sacral chakras that causes a flood of power, creativity and inspiration in a tremendously exciting but somewhat unstable fashion. This is the "in love" phase, where family and friends look on and nod indulgently as the besotted behaves in a quite uncharacteristic fashion. They're temporarily out of control in what's been termed "the purest form of insanity." Often at such times we behave in a way that we would never normally countenance. Contrast this with the creative block and the dearth of activity that occurs as relationships begin to fail.

After its initial opening and flood of hyperactivity, the sacral chakra balances and so the level of sexual activity and the mood also stabilize. This allows a return to normal everyday activity and work, but the connection between the couple remains strong.

Desire, Pleasure and Our Need for Attention

The desire and pleasure that arise at the second chakra are not only of a sensual and sexual nature. Joy in the material as well as the ephemeral helps satisfy us and make us feel complete. The movement is toward incorporating new things, human and material, into our lives. The sense associated with the sacral chakra is that of taste. Go out now and taste and enjoy not only your food but also the world and all it has to offer.

Allowing ourselves to have what we need is a positive move. Unfortunately, understanding our desires and interpreting them correctly sometimes isn't so easy and there can be misunderstandings about what we really do want.

For instance, I may think I want food, but if I stop to examine this I find I'm not hungry at all. Obviously, I have the need for something. Perhaps I'm really bored, or angry, or in pain. There are much more appropriate actions for me to take than eating. Perhaps I need to meditate or go for a walk, or talk through my anger or ask someone to hug me. But because of past conditioning (when I was upset and tearful as a child I may have been given a sweet or an ice cream to pacify me), I now miss out one of the essential cognitive steps and simply go directly to the food rather than look at the cause of my discomfort.

The important thing to recognize is that if you feel you need something, you do. And generally finding what you need and what gives you pleasure has the dual function of satisfying your need and of pointing you in the direction you need to go.

The sacral chakra's desire to both give and receive pleasure is a powerful signpost. If instead of pleasure you keep bumping up against pain, it's very likely you're being encouraged to change direction. Although there's actually no such thing as being in the wrong place or going in the wrong direction, the pain's there to help you learn that you need to move on—a bit like a cattle prod. If you refuse to acknowledge that message, you can find your life going around in circles. It's amazing how often we feel pain and instead of moving out of the way, as we would certainly do with physical pain, we simply redouble our efforts to try overcoming the difficulty.

If you're honest with yourself, how many times have you said, "I'll never let that happen to me again," only to find yourself in a similar place later? How many times have you gotten into the same difficulty in relationships but tried even harder to make it work when all the signals say it's time to go? The sacral chakra is trying to help you with this. If you allow it to open and then listen carefully to its messages, it will generally guide you to steer an accurate course to a happier and healthier way of being. But don't beat yourself up if you still end up in the same place again. Just pause, see what you've learned, then move out of the pain more quickly. You don't have to keep falling down the same hole again and again.

Our need for attention is part of our need to be nurtured. But sometimes, because of early damage, we learn to resort to unusual ways of getting what we need. For some reason, we learn not to ask or to state our needs verbally. Instead we act out our needs and hope that someone will understand. I'm afraid sometimes I still bang doors when I'm very angry. This is called "acting out" behavior and it's often ignored or dismissed, which only leads to escalation in our desperate attempt to be understood. Then there's the horribly pejorative term "attention-seeking behavior." It's much misused and is often a blanket term spat out to cover behavior that's seen as unhealthy and best ignored.

The sad part about this is that attention-seeking behavior is indeed signaling exactly that—someone needs attention, even though they may be asking for it in an unhealthy, distorted and possibly unpleasant way. The effect is totally counterproductive, of course. People who initially try to help eventually feel resentful and exasperated and so withdraw, leaving the person feeling that they must act out their needs with even more gusto since they're still not being heard. If we don't acknowledge that we (and everyone else) both desire and need attention in one form or another, we'll only repress our needs, which will re-emerge elsewhere.

I remember a young man who would come to the emergency room regularly. He'd usually cut himself superficially, but enough to require attention. For a few months this would occur almost on a nightly basis and, as the psychiatrist on duty, I was called to check that he wasn't at risk of killing himself. We developed a good relationship. However, it was obvious to me that here was a sad and lonely boy who had no one to talk to and who used this powerful but dangerous method of communication in order to make someone listen.

Having spent long hours sitting talking to him in the night, I realized that this was actually encouraging his behavior. If he did something as unhealthy and inappropriate as cutting himself, he would be rewarded by being listened to for an hour or so! He wasn't ready to accept proper psychotherapy, so I suggested that as long as I wasn't too busy I'd be happy to see him when I was on call, provided he simply asked. If he cut himself, I wouldn't come.

The next few nights, he came to the hospital, but as usual with superficial lacerations. With some trepidation, I refused to see him and he stormed out. After about a week he came to the hospital and simply asked to see me. We sat and had a long talk, neither of us mentioning the fact that I'd refused to see him on previous occasions, nor that he'd ever cut himself. We'd made a breakthrough.

We began to look at why he needed attention. He was very lonely, living in a squat with two other young men who, like himself, had run away from home. They all used drugs together from time to time, sometimes begging and sometimes stealing for the money to finance their drug habit. What he really needed, and probably they all did, was a home, some nurturing, some mothering and most of all a lot of love. He was stuck. Not only had he no sense of being rooted or of belonging anywhere—a result of the blocking of his root chakra due to the pain he'd had at home in his very early days—but he had very little self-esteem and no idea of his potential as a human being. He was needy and desirous of attention, but he'd found that the only way he would get any at all at home was to be naughty. He would be shouted at or hit, but at least that was something. Now he needed to re-educate himself on several levels.

First, he needed to know that if he spoke instead of screaming and swearing or cutting himself, he was more likely to be heard. Next, even though he might be heard, he wouldn't always get what he wanted and he would have to learn to live with this. And third, he needed to be able to learn to supply some of his needs from within and not always expect that they would come from other people.

The last time I saw him, he was attending college while living in a hostel for young men. He hadn't cut himself or taken drugs for well over a year. What he did during his healing with me was remove the blocks, initially to his sacral chakra and base and thereafter to his throat to help him communicate more healthily. Bit by bit he was able to fill up his core (see Figure 8), which was empty. He needed to fulfill all his needs and desires for love, nurturing and pleasure from outside himself.

We all need love, support, nurturing and touch as well as the basics of food, clothing and shelter. But if we learn to look for all our support from outside, we leave ourselves vulnerable. Filling the central core begins at the root chakra as we develop a sense of self, and continues at the sacral chakra as we find our place within family and community. Providing for our own needs as much as we can from within, but with healthy communication with the outside for what we truly need from there, protects us from vulnerability.

Are You Ready for a Burst of Energy?

As well as governing desire, the sacral chakra also enhances our capacity to retain information, and periods of accelerated learning often accompany its sudden opening. You have much greater potential than you ever believed possible, and work at this chakra primes the solar plexus pump to enable you to achieve it. However, things can start to happen very quickly and you may feel like you're running out of control. But all of this change is for the ultimate good. Soon, you'll realize that you're absorbing knowledge in a way previously impossible, your memory has improved and ready-formed ideas are flooding in as your creativity moves up a notch.

With the opening of the sacral chakra, we begin to feel empowered, paving the way for the fuller development of this power at the solar plexus chakra. We begin in a self-confident rather than conceited way to recognize our gifts and talents, and this allows us to start to see ourselves in our true beauty and magnificence. We begin to feel free of jealousy and greed as we become more comfortable in the knowledge that each of us is unique with a special place and purpose. Initially you may be able only to glimpse this, but as you continue to work on this area and move up to the next chakra, your confidence in your own ability increases.

Even further growth is encouraged as we become more aware that our capabilities are not static but that we're on an ever-increasing growth curve. The work at each chakra is not a once-and-for-all task. We go on refining and improving as our life proceeds, returning again and again to revisit and update our understanding as our spiritual development continues all our earthly lifetime and beyond. You're starting to discover what it's like to be a spiritual being!

Dysfunction at the Sacral Level

If the sacral chakra is sluggish or blocked, there's often an inability to experience orgasm (anorgasmia), a distaste for sex or loss of libido in women and difficulties in maintaining an erection and in ejaculation in men. At the very least, sensual pleasure is harder to achieve. There's a resultant lack of self-confidence and an inability to achieve potential in both sexes.

Since much of the emphasis of this chakra is on movement and flexibility, blocking will often result in stiffness and a lack of graceful

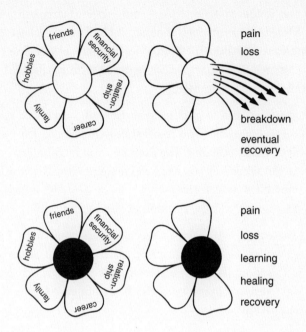

Figure 8: *In 8a, let us imagine that this person is supported by family, friends, career, a rela-tionship and financial security. However, there is little if any inner strength—her core is empty. Should any one of those supports be lost, let us say for example that her husband leaves her and with him goes her financial security, it is unlikely that she'll be able to deal well with the loss. There's a possibility of a "breakdown" until inner resources have been found to allow for stability to be established again.*

In 8b, the person here has exactly the same supportive relationships with family, friends, career, etc., but she also has a strong sense of self, good self-esteem and self-confidence: a strong core. Should any of her external supports be lost, she will of course suffer grief, but she has inner strength to deal with this and to survive without breakdown.

movement, particularly in the lower back, hips and legs. Everything seems to be clogged up, and flow (there's that word again) seems to be lost on all levels. Stasis in the urinary tract can clog up your waterworks and result in fluid retention, recurrent cystitis, infections, kidney stones, nephritis and other such problems. Blocked lymph vessels can cause swelling and tender spots on ankles and legs and circulation is not at its best. Menstrual problems abound, including premenstrual syndrome, increased tension, irritability and anxiety as swelling compromises the tissues. Irregular periods with or without heavy bleeding and clotting are fairly common.

Everything from mood to muscles feels tight and rigid and relaxation is almost impossible since you're constantly defensive. How exhausting! However, help is at hand. The exercises and meditations are going to help you, but wherever you are, keep remembering the word "flow." Say it to yourself slowly, feeling what it means, and let it happen. Just let yourself flow, physically, emotionally and spiritually.

I worked for a good while with a woman who came along to see me with huge swollen legs, her skin stretched and painful as she shuffled stiffly into the room. In her mid-forties, she looked much older and was having a variety of problems. Her body appeared quite rigid and she had painful stiff joints.

She was depressed beyond tears and with a sad resignation she responded to my questioning about her childhood. Her father had wanted a boy, she said, and she was always aware of what a disappointment she'd been to him. He'd criticized her mercilessly and her first few years at school had been torture as she'd tried to be athletic and do well while feeling constantly in conflict with that part of her that wanted to be soft, feminine and girlish. Whatever she did, she couldn't seem to please him, and bit by bit she'd given up trying. In doing so, she still couldn't allow herself to enjoy growing into adolescence and womanhood. She had never enjoyed sex and although she'd eventually married, it had been a joyless affair which had come to an end when her husband found a mate more to his liking.

Since then she had lived alone as her physical health continued to deteriorate. She'd lost sight, if ever she had it, of who she really was and now expected nothing from life. Even in coming to see me she kept apologizing for the fact that I probably wouldn't be able to help her.

She had a completely blocked sacral chakra with resultant stasis throughout her body. Her physical as well as emotional energy was low and the initial work was simply to get things moving and to over-come her resistance, which was as rigid as her body. Bit by bit she began to shift the block as we worked on clearing the pain of the past, which she'd almost forgotten and certainly felt was totally uncon-nected to her current problems. She was astounded when some weeks later she had a previously unknown flutter in her psyche and recog-nized it as a sexual urge. The swelling and stiffness were beginning to subside and she was able, quite self-consciously at first, to try some of the exercises at the end of this chapter. I'm happy to say that she was eventually able to let go of that long-buried pain and to allow her fem-ininity to develop. With it came her creativity and as she poured out poetry that bathed and healed her soul, we were able to conclude our sessions together as she took over her own healing.

No single chakra can exist in isolation and when the floodgates of the water-based sacral center are opened, the force is great enough to move anything in its path and blocks at other levels can begin to melt away also. As the charisma of the first chakra now leads into the sec-ond and we glimpse real possibilities, the faint-hearted may pause or halt. But it's at this point that our lives can move on a trajectory which we could never have envisaged. We're now setting a course to abun-dance and prosperity. Fed by the earth, the energy is transmuted through the root chakra and empowered by the second before moving up to be further refined at the third. Harnessing this energy is imper-ative if we're to control and use it to the full.

However, a word of warning. Ego can completely diffuse the poten-tial that's now about to be released. The power we're just touching, and can feel growing and pushing up through our physical as well as mental and spiritual bodies, is of a truly spiritual nature and must be used for the good of all. Any attempt to misuse it here will result in calamity. The potential of the sacral needs to be tempered with the conscience and love of the higher centers to gain its maximum force. If we truly use this with pure heart and good intention, we're ready to receive the abundance that's promised by the solar plexus.

The right to make our own choices and decisions is part of the chal-lenge of the earthly life, and at this point we can choose a course set for growth and accomplishment, abundance and power in its most loving and spiritual sense, or lose what's now at our fingertips.

The following exercises and meditations will help you to achieve your goals as you clear and gently open the sacral chakra.

The Exercises

Exercise 1

Play some music that's gentle and flowing and reminds you of water. There are some lovely pieces to choose from, but if you have difficulty in finding one, I've made a list of some of my favorites in Chapter 8 (pages 174–76).

Give yourself as much space as you can and wear something that's not restricting. Gently begin to move with the music. Just let your body move where it wishes as tension starts to be released. Allow your body to relax and become more flexible. Feel your natural grace start to emerge. Feel as though you are flowing with the water, moving gently. Maybe so far your feet have remained still on the ground. If so, perhaps you could gently begin to move them. Take your time. Flow. Move. Let go of any pain or tension. Breathe into it. Allow there to be harmony and gentle flow. Move. Be aware of the sensations in your body. You are fully aware. You are allowing your creativity to open as you gently sway. Release emotions as they arise. Just let them go. Gently, gently, move with the music. Allow yourself to begin to get lost in the music. Allow the movement to create change in your life. Allow there to be a new rhythm to life. Flow. Be flexible. Flexible in your joints, flexible in your attitudes, flexible in your approach to life. Move. Flow. Become part of the music. Allow yourself to be. Enjoy.

When the music ends, take your time to become still. Remain with your eyes closed for a few moments until you feel reoriented. Gently resume a relaxed pose. When you are ready and fully grounded back in the room, open your eyes. Gently stretch your joints while affirming that you are becoming more and more flexible. Have a drink of clear energized water (see page 26).

Exercise 2

Make yourself a bath or prepare a shower. Light a candle where it will be safe. If you're taking a bath, use some essential oils (rosemary or amber would be good). If you're taking a shower, use a vaporizer to scent the atmosphere or burn some incense. Now, take your time and as you soak in the water, affirm that you are allowing the water to wash away anything negative, to cleanse you of impurity and to release anything that is now outdated and needs to be discarded. When you are ready, gently cleanse your skin, making long strokes down your long bones and circular movements over your joints. As you do so, affirm that you are becoming more flexible, that your joints are free. Feel the internal movement also and feel the flow of the fluids within your body. Affirm that you are letting go of any fluid you don't need, that your bodily fluids are flowing freely, that the fluid in your body is clear and clean and bathing your cells. Allow yourself to feel nurtured as you now massage your body, gently but firmly . . . long movement over bones, circular movements over joints . . . and otherwise following the flow of your skin. Love yourself. Affirm that you are becoming more healthy and free. Take as long as you wish.

When you are finished wrap yourself in warm towels or a warm robe. Relax and have a long drink of energized water.

Exercise 3

The sacral chakra is associated with the sense of taste. When you prepare your food or have something to drink, spend a moment initially preparing to taste it fully. Eat slowly, enjoying each bite. Know that the food is giving you its energy. Raw live foods such as vegetables and salad are imparting their energy and increasing your vitality. The water you drink is cleansing you. If you take energized water, the energy of the crystal is also stimulating you. Enjoy your sense of taste.

The Meditations

Meditation 1

Choose a time when you won't be disturbed for at least an hour so that you have adequate time not only for the meditation, but also to be alone and quiet for a while afterward if that's what you need. As always, take yourself to your safe place if you can, or find a place by some water where you will be safe and can relax completely.

Crystals that would be useful are moonstone or topaz. Moonstone is not only good at balancing your emotions but has a particular effect on fertility, menstrual cramps and premenstrual syndrome. It also increases flexibility and is very nurturing. Topaz is wonderful for almost everything! It is another stone along with amethyst that I wear almost every day, especially when I'm working. It's soothing and peaceful and yet gives a boost to creativity, while being quite powerful at aiding healing and regeneration.

You need to be able to sit with your spine erect if you can, but most importantly choose a position you can hold. If you need the support of a chair, use it; if you'd prefer cushions, that's fine too.

FORGIVING THE PAST

As always, begin by focusing on your breathing the way you did in the last meditation and allow yourself to relax. Know that you are in a safe place. You're protected and grounded.

You're going to heal and let go of anything that happened to you between the ages of about three to five and eight. Allow yourself to encompass that time in your life. Whatever happened is a memory now—you've already survived. All that's needed now is for you to let it go so that it doesn't prevent you from living your life to the full. Without spending time on the details, gather together the events of that time into a parcel so you can heal them.

In your heart wrap your child self in love and compassion, holding and protecting tenderly and securely.

Now, with a thought, send out healing and forgiveness to that time, to those events and if possible to the people of then. Let light shine around and through all of it so it can be healed and you can be free. Particularly send love and healing to your child self. Hold that part of you with great compassion. Love your child self.

And now, if you are able, you can move to the second stage.

Move to a spiritual perspective and look at the people, the events and the energies of that time. Perhaps you can see that the people of that time did what they did because of their own damage and their own pain. If you can, send them compassion. And, if you can, forgive them and in doing so set yourself free of them for good. Let it go. You can be free . . . forgive.

Take your time.

And now, if you are able, move to the third stage.

Move to a higher spiritual perspective and look again. Maybe now you can see that the events that occurred then were moving you through your life's lessons and teaching you things you needed to know to be more whole. In the totality of your spiritual life there needed to be teachers so you could learn. If you are able, allow yourself to see those who were involved in your process at that time as those who gave you the experience you needed and, if you can, thank them and set them free.

Take your time. Give thanks.

Feel your child self with a different sense of peace and serenity. Allow yourself to feel whole and very gently start to return to your physical self. Feel your feet on the ground. Be aware of your physical body and its strong connection with the earth. Hold your physical body, and when you feel present behind your eyes, very gently open them. When you are ready, stretch. And, when you are ready, move.

Have a drink of water and record whatever you wish in your notebook.

Meditation 2

Using the same technique, get into that comfortable and relaxed space within yourself. Now, take your focus down through your heart chakra, down through your solar plexus and to the sacral chakra. See a beautiful orange light there. Allow yourself to wonder at its beauty—shining, swirling light, full of energy, radiant energy. Watch it swirling. Now allow yourself to gently enter it, into the orange light, feel its radiance, feel its warmth, feel its energy. Allow yourself to move gently through the light with a sense of delight at being able to explore. Allow yourself to be carried gently along and you will find that you are moving out through the light and into clear beautiful water. Feel the water gently flowing around you. You are able to breathe quite easily. Everything is gently flowing. Feel the water soft on your skin, feel it gently massage your body as it flows around you. Gently, gently, flowing. Gently flowing. Allow yourself to be carried along. Enjoy the feeling. See how effortlessly you move in the water.

Move wherever you wish. Feel your body light and flexible. Your body moves like the water, flowing, gently flowing, supple, lithe, flowing, gently flowing.

Explore as much as you want to. This is a beautiful serene place. Feel its peace, feel its beauty. Take your time.

In a moment, look to the right and you will be delighted to see, approaching you through the water, a beautiful, powerful yet gentle being. You perceive its power, its magnificence, its vitality and its strong love for you. Watch it as it approaches you. Send out a loving, welcoming thought to it. Feel its stimulating energy as it approaches. This is your masculine principle. Enjoy it. Touch it, welcome it, befriend it. Feel its presence, its benevolence, its beauty, its protection. Feel its power as it comes alongside you. Enjoy. Send out a loving message to it.

And now gaze off to your left and you will see another being approaching. This one is soft and gentle, beautiful and loving but with strength and wisdom in its vulnerability. You perceive its radiance and its benevolent power. You feel its loving passion, its mysterious beauty, its magnificence. Feel its love for you, deep and passionate. Watch it, hold it in your gaze. Send a warm, loving, welcoming thought to it, for this is your feminine principle. Enjoy it, its gentleness, its power, its serenity. Welcome it. Touch it, befriend it. Watch its graceful movement. Allow it to come alongside you. Send a loving message out to it.

And now, as you watch, the two move out together, entering into a wonderful graceful swirling dance. They move together, flowing around and into each other, swirling, blending, moving apart and then rejoining each other, uniting in wholeness and perfection. Watch them as they move. Feel the water, feel their love for each other and their love for you, feel the water filled with love and joy, feel their vitality, their creativity, their harmony, their balance. And now, they are beckoning you. Come, you are drawn toward them and mingle and blend with them. You are taken up in their wondrous dance. You move with them and unite with them. You feel your beauty, feel your magnificence. Feel your power. Feel your wholeness. Enjoy.

Feel all the flowing fluid within you. Let there be gentle, steady flow within as well as around you. Feel your circulation, free and easily flowing. Feel the fluid circulating in your tissues. Feel the cleansing and healing of the water, gently cleansing, healing and balancing. Healing and balancing, gently flowing. Feel the flowing movement of your body, the flexibility of your movement, the freedom you move with. Feel yourself nurtured. Let yourself receive. Feel the pleasure of being nurtured. Enjoy.

And now feeling whole, with your masculine and your feminine in harmony and balance, with freedom and serenity, allow yourself to prepare to return, gently. Take your time. Move back toward the light, the orange light, moving gently toward it, now, entering it. Moving gently through its brilliance, you find yourself moving back out through your sacral chakra, gently, gently.

Bring your focus gently back to your physical presence, gently back to the room, gently back to this point in time. Gently. When you feel that you are back somewhere behind your eyes, keeping your eyes closed, feel your physical presence. Feel your feet on the ground. Move your toes. Feel your connection with the earth. Hold your physical body and, when you are ready, but only then, gently open your eyes. Gently open your eyes and be present and grounded. Stay where you are for a moment. Feel your grounding and when you are ready, stretch and move.

Have a drink of water and record whatever you wish in your notebook.

SIX

The Solar Plexus:
Power, Will and Prosperity

∾

I dedicate my life to the power within me.
Through dedication I unfold naturally to the
highest potential of my being.
This is my day.
I control each and every thing that comes to me.
I accept complete responsibility for my life.
I am power.
So be it.

Please read the above quotation again. Slowly. Savor every word. All of the power of the solar plexus is represented here. This could be its voice. "I am power." "Through dedication I unfold naturally to the highest potential of my being."

Just feel these words. Say them again and feel your whole being move. Say them slowly. This is the solar plexus. It's a magical chakra. Being a Leo and ruled by the sun, the solar plexus, my own personal sun, is perhaps one of my favorite chakras. The chakra of fire, it glows golden yellow radiating our fire out into the world.

Occupying the area between the lower chest and the navel, the solar plexus moves us from the base material world to the ephemeral. As we make the transition toward the mental and intellectual, it offers us a potent concoction of passion and energy, laced with opinion and logic, motivation and drive. The work at the first and second chakras has primed the pump, the solidity of the root giving rise to the flowing movement of the sacral chakra. Now we stand at the threshold of enormous change as we build on the ideas that have emerged. The pleasure/pain principle of the second chakra is a useful signpost to indicate our way forward, but the choice to create our own life strategy in whatever way we wish comes now. The solar plexus offers us liberation. It's up to us whether we take it.

It's time for action, for taking charge, for deciding upon our course. All is ready for each of us to capture and harness our will, to be dynamic, and with motivation and drive, to move forward. Though communication and self-expression are functions of the throat chakra, it's here at the solar plexus that our opinions are formed. It's here that we develop the courage to express ourselves in the world as our truth emerges. We discover our own inner strength and freedom and we develop the tenacity to keep going despite difficult life events and circumstances. We now have the will to achieve and succeed as we radiate our energy and become a force to be reckoned with. We have arrived, and the world needs to know that we are here.

Well utilized, the power of the solar plexus gives us unlimited possibilities—to work, to create change, to become what we want to be, to realize our ambitions, to be happy, to drive our lives wherever we want to go. Misused, this heady commodity can become a dangerous weapon we can wield over others, insensitively riding rough-shod over the sensibilities of those who are less in touch with their own power. This is simply the road to eventual disaster.

Our journey has brought us to the seat of our personality, the foundation of our own personal identity. It's often the work at this chakra that produces the most fireworks in our ascent as we let go of old pent-up emotion and unspent feelings, so hold on to your hat. But if we do the work here, we transform ourselves and our lives. We can move toward peace and contentment with ourselves and the world in a way we've probably never known before.

Recognizing Our Power

When I'm teaching about the chakras, I usually start with a quick sketch of the whole system. When I get to the solar plexus, the powerhouse of the chakra system, I always feel my own power move. I see my physical movements and my posture change. My breathing alters as I allow the essence of the solar plexus to be expressed. Usually, I keep my power well under wraps since I know it can be intimidating (we'll talk more about this later), but I can't really express this most amazing of chakras without addressing its power.

If ever I feel that life has been unfair (yes, I do feel that sometimes), it's my solar plexus I go to. I cup it in my hands and let it start to whisper its power. Slowly, and feeling every word, I let it gently unfold. I am the power. I begin to have a physical sensation at the solar plexus. I am the power. It starts to grow and I unfurl to my full height. I am the power. The energy starts to trickle and soon becomes a flood. I am the power. I open my chest and my shoulders. I am the power. My chin comes up and my shoulders fall. I am the power. My head tilts back and my face lifts upward. I am the power. My arms move out now away from my solar plexus and my hands reach up to the sky. I am the power. My voice is stronger now and even if I don't open my throat and use it to the full, I know how it will sound. I am the power. I am now powerful but peaceful. I can face anything. I can overcome anything. I can be all that I need to be. I can learn all that I need to learn. I am responsible for me and no one can ever take that away from me no matter what they do to me. I am powerful. My solar plexus is clear and strong. I am in control of me and what happens to me. I am the power. I accept responsibility for my life. So be it.

It feels wonderful. Within minutes I can be back in control and out of what could otherwise become an attack of the "poor me" syndrome.

Recognizing the power in all of us is one of the most liberating things we can do. No longer do we see ourselves as victims, unable to change our circumstances. At last we begin to take responsibility for having gotten where we are, good or bad, and with this comes the certainty that we can also move ourselves into a different and better place. Isn't that wonderful? We can actually make our lives happen. We can get into the driving seat and steer a course of our choice. It really is up to us. But what a responsibility. It sounds inviting, but are you really ready for it? No more blaming someone else for what happens to you. No more abdicating responsibility. My life is mine and mine alone. It's up to me to live it my way.

Hapless Victim to Victorious Survivor

The solar plexus is the home of our will—our ability to make things happen because we will them to be so. Provided we have a pure heart and good intention to do something for the benefit of all (including ourselves) we are able to manifest most things in our lives. The amazing force produced by a combination of our power and will makes us capable of more than we ever imagined. The greatest power of all, of course, is love. It has amazing effects on our lives. Acting for everyone's higher good is love. It's love combined with power and will that makes wonderful things happen. Go back and read the quotation at the beginning of the chapter again.

> I control each and every thing that comes to me.
> I accept complete responsibility for my life.
> I am power.
> So be it.

What an affirmation. Why not copy that out and put it in all the places where you can see it often and see what starts to happen to your life.

Sometimes we haven't used our power wisely and we may not like the results of the choices we've made, but if we begin to own our mistakes, we're in a position to change our actions and produce a different outcome. If we've rendered ourselves apparently helpless, we did it using our power and our will in a way that wasn't useful to us. We haven't necessarily used it wrongly, but the choices we've made have led us to something other than that which we really want. You can just as easily will something good into your life.

If you feel that you have very little, just look around you. We all have more than we appreciate. But it may be that some of the things you have, you no longer want. You may prefer to change them for something different or better. You can do that.

One woman, with whom I worked for quite a long time, eventually came to a workshop. She'd suffered some nasty life events and had been stripped of much that she possessed. One of the affirmations I often use in my workshops is "I have all that I need and more." She says she had a mixture of laughter and tears while trying to repeat this silently in meditation. However, after a while, it became one of the most comforting things she could say to herself. If she looked at possessions and material wealth, she certainly had much less. However, in terms of support, friendship and love, she really did have all she needed and more. She says her life began to change as soon as she started to redefine her values and use the affirmation regularly. But accepting that right now we have all we need and more doesn't mean there aren't more wonderful things to come.

Obviously, there are some circumstances that appear to be beyond our control, not born of any conscious or unconscious action on our part. Some of the people I work with have suffered horrendous abuse, trauma and deprivation. Although in adulthood they may continue to perpetuate the only way of life they know, for example, by continuing to put themselves in abusive situations, neither as children nor as adults do they deserve what happens to them. Those of us who have the enormous privilege of working closely with such souls in torment need to learn well what they are teaching us.

It's been said that souls reaching their completion and almost ready to return to the body of God will often set themselves very heavy and painful tasks to complete in this lifetime. In time, we may see all life events as valuable lessons in the immense scheme of things, suffered by wise, ancient spirits in order to complete their learning. Perhaps they're here to work out not only their own karma (see Glossary) but to generously carry some of the karma of humanity in general. In doing so, they bring to the attention of the world what we need to see and change. For example, children who are born in areas in the world where there's great poverty or deprivation and who are only here for days, weeks or months are souls sacrificing themselves to physical misery for a very short period to highlight the plight of the many who live constantly in hunger or disease. The same can be said of other children who come very briefly to teach their parents, perhaps the doctors and others something they need to learn.

This doesn't mean that only those in pain are great ancient souls nor that pain indicates an ancient spirit. There are many young souls who have much to learn who are working things out in a very painful manner. There are others who are repaying karmic debts (see Glossary). In this lifetime, they don't move much closer toward enlightenment since their agenda is to work only on the pain. And there are wise, ancient, peaceful souls who have done much of their own work and are now here to teach and give and thereby to continue their own growth. All are powerful and each is exercising their human will in living the earthly life before returning home to the freedom of the spiritual.

Some people are not hapless victims at all but give the appearance of helplessness because it suits them to do so. Sometimes they are among the strongest around. There are many secondary gains for those who are "helpless" (as there are for those who are willing to play the rescue game): for example, they are relieved of taking responsibility for their lives, using others to do things for them that they could well do for themselves. But they stunt their growth by doing so, and there are other negative consequences.

Betty and Rich were one such "victim and rescuer" couple. They presented together, only because Rich felt he had to bring Betty along to make sure she got to my consulting room safely and that she remembered to tell me all that was wrong with her. Each time I asked her a question, he answered, and even when I gently suggested that I'd like

RELATIONSHIPS

Although the heart chakra deals with human loving (see Chapter 7), it is at the level of the solar plexus that we become strong and stable enough to be able to enter into long-term relationships and make them work. Deeply bonding with another demands that the solar plexus be open along with the heart. However, this makes the ending of relationships doubly painful, as we not only disentangle the heart cords that have bound us, but also sever the solar plexus attachment.

The solar plexus also allows us to have a sense of home, of commitment and belonging. It is where our sense of patriotism and our qualities of consistency and loyalty reside.

to hear her version, Betty sought his approval with a glance before she attempted to answer. Rich's concern for her was very real and his love for her genuine. However, they were both caught in different aspects of the solar plexus game. She was "helpless" and he was taking care of the situation. Her gains were that she didn't need to take responsibility for herself, and his that he had her never-ending devotion.

This is the co-dependent relationship I mentioned in Chapter 5 and will talk about again in Chapter 7. There are issues for every chakra here. Betty could, with a single glance, control Rich—such was her power. In her "helplessness" she was the victor. But similarly, Rich could continue to control her by refusing to let her do anything for herself, constantly sending both verbal and non-verbal messages that she wasn't strong enough to cope without him. Such is the damaged solar plexus. Both had baggage they'd brought to the relationship and had never sorted. It was wonderful to see them grow together as they began to tell each other the whole truth for the first time, each witnessing the other clearing old hurt, letting it go and getting free. Both grew in stature as they now had good healthy gain from being well and being together. We had an amazing time on the first day that Betty was able to say she disagreed and was angry, rather than retreating to her bed as she might have in the past. It was time for me to go and let them get on with it.

Being independent and responsible brings rewards that far outweigh dependence-driven gains. Such rewards include self-realization and with it, the confidence, courage and responsibility to stand up and be counted for who we are. It brings a feeling of excitement that gives way to a new inner peace and harmony. Life is becoming easier. We start to realize we can make our life happen.

Pride in Our Individuality

With the opening of the solar plexus chakra comes the development of self-respect and with it, a growing ability to respect others for who they are. We come to appreciate diversity as a gift and a challenge that enriches us all. We learn to adapt and accommodate difference and refine our opinions and beliefs. Being willing to bend a little and compromise if necessary combines the mighty oak with the pliable willow and ensures easy progress and development.

As our capacity to integrate and cooperate with others is enhanced, there is a developing joy in exploring the new and different. We begin to have pride in our individuality but within the context of a balanced totality. Previously, we may have felt separation and isolation but now there's a recognition of being simultaneously complete and yet part of a greater whole. Wisdom born of experience walks hand in hand with humility as we see ourselves powerful at the center of our universe and yet a tiny speck in the great scheme of things.

We now come into balance not only with all of humanity but with nature and all of the universe. In the past we may have responded to authority or those we have perceived as being in power by feeling either small and insignificant or, conversely, rebellious, superior and aggressive. From the standpoint of equality we can now see both attitudes as similarly inappropriate. Though we've learned to value others, their opinions and their contribution to life, we're aware that we no longer need to stand alienated and alone or feel inferior. Having such self-assurance enables us to work alongside others as a team while retaining our individual identity. We know that we all have something unique to offer to every situation.

Live Well and Prosper

Nature is in continuous cyclical motion—the ebb and flow of the tides, the changing of the seasons, the passage of time from day to night, the lunar and menstrual cycles and the spinning of the planets. The solar plexus begs us to respect this need for motion to keep the river of energy flowing. We can do this by radiating our power and light into the world while being open to receive its gifts.

When I am open to receive, I visualize myself gently opening somewhere in the region of my chest and I get a warm, quickening feeling and a particular physical sensation between my heart and my solar plexus (rather vague, I know, but it's hard to describe accurately). I affirm that I am open to receive the abundance of the universe and any opportunities that are for my ultimate good. I send a loving thought up to the heavens and then let it go with absolute confidence that what I need will come flowing into my life very shortly. The results are often miraculous, sometimes not at all what I would have expected and usually, in retrospect, far more than I could have envisaged anyway.

The board outside a local community hall I recently saw read, "If your ship hasn't come in yet, why not row out to meet it?" Doing work on our prosperity is like that. We can sit and wait for something to happen, and grumble that it hasn't, but if we're wise, we can take control and go out and meet it halfway and make it happen. There's absolutely nothing wrong with being prosperous. In fact, I think we have a duty to do all we can to prosper, since in doing so we can keep the river of energy flowing through the universe so that everyone benefits. However, the universal rule is that we must give first in order to receive.

Imagine now that you are looking at the water system at home. Water fills the tank and sits there doing nothing until you turn on a tap. Then there's flow that makes room for some more water to flow in. If you don't open the tap, there's stagnation. No more water can flow in. Your life can get like that. You may keep the tap closed, hoarding what you already have, but in doing that you block new and exciting possibilities in the form of energy, possessions, love, work, etc.

But remembering the "give to receive" rule, we need to be willing to gently push the cycle of prosperity if we want it to work for us. If we do so by giving first, we're rewarded with prosperity on all levels—in work, love, peace, material wealth,

There are many who appear to be prosperous, you may say, but who don't obey that law. But prosperity is not only measured in terms of financial security. I dare say if you looked in all the areas previously mentioned you'd find that they may not be so prosperous after all. It's of scarce value to have lots of money but little peace of mind, or be

DIGESTIVE FIRE

The digestive symptoms that parallel events in relationships (for example the lack of desire for food or voracious appetite in the early stages of falling in love and the nausea, inability to eat and the feeling of being hit in the stomach when there's hurt or betrayal in a bonded relationship) are due to the solar plexus and its association with digestion and the whole abdominal area.

Remember that this is the chakra of fire. The solar plexus governs our digestive processes, allowing for the physical combustion of our food to release energy in a form we can readily use. It is this digestive fire that gives us feelings of hunger when it's high, urging us to refuel our bodies. If we learn to tune in to it, we can eat when it's at its highest (usually at midday when solar energy is at its highest), when it will then burn our food efficiently, releasing all the energy available and leaving little waste to be stored as fat. Then when the digestive fire is low we can eat little, if at all, since our body is telling us it doesn't need to be refueled at present. Listening to this simple signal can help us to maintain weight balance.

flooded with work and not take time to enjoy the benefits of your labor. A healthy solar plexus opens our way to true prosperity.

Blocks at the Solar Plexus

Certain emotions are called "negative" because we don't like to feel them. They include anger, rage, jealousy, resentment and guilt. They are, however, very potent movers in our lives if we allow ourselves to experience them. If, for some reason, we haven't dealt with them, it's at the solar plexus that they get stuck.

The development of the solar plexus begins at about the age of eight or nine, so trauma or distress at this age can have a marked effect on us. Generally, the earlier the trauma and the more it has hurt, the more likely we are to put a lid on it. "Repression" is the psychological term. Sometimes we become so good at this that we're no longer aware of its existence.

I frequently see people who have no memory at all of their childhood, which often turns out to have been pretty grim. As you start the work at the solar plexus, you may be afraid of releasing your feelings lest they erupt like a volcano, destroying yourself and everything around you. The good news is that if we proceed with care, it doesn't have to be destructive. If we harness the heat of rage, for example, we can use it as fuel to rocket us forth healthily. Often it's anger or hate that catapults us out of dying relationships, abusive situations and outdated habits. It allows us to distance ourselves enough not to get tangled up in the emotion or manipulation that has shackled us for too long.

If this chakra is out of balance or blocked we feel like frustrated victims of circumstance, our feelings repressed, our confidence sapped and our integrity compromised. Complaints of tiredness, low energy and poor stamina are common and we may find our desires thwarted as we try to move forward. Without the energy and momentum that a healthy solar plexus gives us, life becomes a great effort, exhausting us at every turn as we constantly meet with resistance. We appear weak-willed, lacking self-determination, self-expression and direction.

Drive and motivation are also affected as we studiously avoid any situation that may prompt a crisis and risk the release of the fear and pain we're trying to hide.

The sad thing is that blocking emotion can be so effective that the good stuff is also cut off. Love and joy, so necessary to inspire and give strength, are lost to us when we're in desperate need of both.

There's often a desperate kind of emotional wandering. Many find difficulty with commitment and form flimsy attachments from need rather than on the basis of love. Because no one gets to really know these people, they're deprived of the validation they so earnestly desire.

As the emotional and spiritual self is blocked, so is the physical. The digestive system rebels with indigestion, ulcers, acidity, constipation, irritable bowel syndrome, diverticulosis and other chronic bowel and digestive disorders. Constipation may alternate with periods of diarrhea. (My doctor self needs to say here that if you have such a pattern of alternating constipation and diarrhea, please go to your general practitioner and have it checked out.)

Since the pancreas is governed by the solar plexus, diabetes mellitus may also occur. The gall bladder and bile ducts may become blocked with the development of stones, and abdominal discomfort aggravates the picture. Eating in a vain and maladaptive attempt to find comfort may cause further complications. The already compromised digestive system is overloaded, adding to its already considerable difficulties. Obesity further lowers self-esteem.

The association between repressed anger and the development of cancer has been well documented. Symptoms of stress abound, including irritability, disturbed sleep, lack of enthusiasm, fatigue, weight gain or loss, depression and sometimes feelings of despair. Does any of that sound familiar?

The picture is one of stagnation on all levels often alternating with overflow—there is either little emotion, or it floods out without control; little motivation to do anything with an occasional burst of energy leading to over-tiredness and fatigue; the unwillingness to be self-assertive and say what needs to be said, and then an occasional outburst with many truths being spoken, but in an aggressive and inappropriate fashion.

Since flow in the central channel is blocked between the upper and lower chakras, there is often coldness of the pelvis and lower limbs, with poor circulation and stiffness. Doing the work necessary to clear and harmonize our energy at this point releases us to move physically, emotionally and spiritually with strength of will, with power, clarity, self-assertion and purpose. Old arthritic pain may improve considerably when the solar plexus has been cleared and freed.

When the solar plexus is too open, however, we often find ourselves picking up other people's negative energy and emotion. In particular we can absorb anger and disquiet.

Closing At Will

Those who behave in a willful and foolhardy manner, using their power with total disregard for others, riding rough-shod over others' feelings without a thought, usually have a solar plexus problem. They exhibit little sensitivity or self-discipline. They show little respect for other people's (or society's) boundaries, either physical, emotional or psychological. These people can wreak havoc not only in their own lives but also in the lives of those they come into contact with. This is

GUT FEELINGS

The solar plexus is where our "gut feelings" reside. It's the raw stuff of our intuition, which reappears in a much more refined form in the sixth chakra, the brow. But as we begin to tune in to our intuition here, preparing for it to be honed to perfection at that higher level, we begin to learn to trust it, to appreciate having at our fingertips an extra, highly accurate sense that can guide us more surely than the other five when it comes to issues of truth, integrity and behavior. So accurate can the sensors of the solar plexus be that it has been termed the second brain.

often the presentation of the condition that has been labeled socio-pathic personality disorder.

Please have compassion for those who behave in this way. If the solar plexus is stuck and has not been cleared of the anger, rage and pain that are compacted there, there's often little that person can do to prevent the eruption of the mess that they would desperately like to hide. The same holds true if their repression has become weak, which sometimes happens as we get older or if there is a life event powerful enough to catch us off our guard and lift the lid. They need courage and help clearing the old emotion, though such catharsis (see Glossary) will only be of lasting value if there's simultaneous healing in the space where the pain has been stored. Though we need to be able to shut down on all levels (except the root, which should always be open to keep us grounded), nowhere is this so important as it is at the solar plexus, since the energy we can pick up here can be the most negative and damaging.

I have a patient who works with a colleague who is angry and immature and has little respect for others, often hurling verbal abuse as well as objects. My patient needed to learn to close his solar plexus very tightly before going to work since otherwise he not only finds himself feeling exhausted and battered, but also he carries much of the anger home and dumps it on his family. Eventually he may learn not to allow himself to be in such an abusive situation. But for the present, he doesn't have to pick up the negativity that he's surrounded by on a daily basis—and neither do others in his family. He uses the following exercise to close his solar plexus and protect himself.

As a quick thirty-second first aid, imagine there's a beautiful yellow flower at your solar plexus with its petals fully open. Then, with your eyes closed, visualize it closing up into a very tight bud. You'll be amazed at how you'll stop picking up emotional and psychological junk.

Closing the solar plexus at will needs practice and it's worth checking several times a day if necessary to see that you're not wide open to everyone else's mess.

Ready for a Change?

Now is the time for you to start making new choices. You can use your power reinforced by your considered will to make healthy changes that can become permanent if you want them to be.

What you need to do as a first step is to

- acknowledge your innate power
- have a look at what you really want
- with thought, discipline and control, actively exercise your will to direct your life in the way you choose
- be fair, just, honest and sensitive to yourself and others

Sound easy? It can be if you approach it with a positive attitude, with confidence and with an eye on your purpose. As always, remember that whatever comes up while you are doing the work is only memory. You have already survived.

The Exercises

Exercise 1

Write a letter that you're not going to send to each of your parents. In this letter you're able to say anything and everything you ever wanted to say to them but never could. Or it may be that you've said these things before but feel you weren't heard. You don't have to censor what you want to say in any way, because no one ever needs to see the letters except you. You can swear if you wish, you can scream and shout. It all goes into the letter. When you feel it's complete, leave it where you have good access to it (though preferably somewhere others don't) so you can add to it over the next day or so if you want to.

When you feel it's really finished, end it in whatever way you feel you can. If you can say that both you and your parents are released from anything either of you did to hurt the other and forgive, that would be wonderful, but if you're not ready to do that, don't worry.

Seal the letter in an envelope and leave it for at least a week before you open it and reread it. You may never want to do so. That's okay. You can either ceremonially burn it or destroy it in some other way, or keep it somewhere very safe to destroy when you are ready.

Now take a lovely bath or shower to cleanse you from the past so that you can let it go (oils for your bath or vaporizer could include rose or ylang-ylang).

Exercise 2

Go to your safe place and arrange a seat for yourself and an empty seat close by where you can see it. Close your eyes for a moment and bring to mind your child self of nine or ten years old. Allow the child to go and sit on the other chair. Let your child self tell you what has been happening to her/him lately. Listen quietly and attentively, and with love and compassion. When s/he has finished, respond in whatever way you feel is appropriate, with love and compassion. Does the child need a hug? Does s/he need praise? Does s/he need encouragement? The last thing s/he needs is judgement, chastising, hitting or punishment of any kind. Most of all s/he needs to be told that s/he is loved and cherished and that you will never abandon her/him. Take your time. Be calm and patient. Love yourself, love your child self. When you are ready, allow your child self to return to your heart where s/he belongs. Welcome your child home. Do your grounding exercise (see page 78). Be gentle with yourself. Take some time for you and then write up in your journal whatever you wish.

Exercise 3

Starting with the following affirmations as a guide, adjust them bit by bit until they feel just right for you. Then write them on cards to put in prominent places where you'll see them regularly. (My favorite place is always the fridge door. I'm certainly going to be there several times most days.)

- I open my heart and mind to receive the power of the universe, which I use for my higher good and the higher good of all.

- I welcome opportunities to fulfill my highest potential.

- I am responsible for me, my health, my welfare and my behavior. I accept this with gratitude.

- I use my will to create the best possible life for myself and others.

- I am open to receive prosperity in all its forms.

If you really want the affirmations to work for you, remember you need to work at them!

The Meditations

Meditation 1

Go to your safe place and make sure you won't be disturbed for at least an hour. Have your crystal close by. Here again, topaz would be good, but my favorite for the solar plexus is citrine. This is sometimes called the "abundance stone" which stimulates personal power, prosperity and creativity. It also brings cheerfulness, hope and positivity. What could be better for this chakra?

If you have a yellow flower then have that close by, but otherwise anything yellow will do. Light your candle, making sure it will be safe while you have your eyes closed. Take the phone off the hook.

Using the usual method of achieving a relaxed state, get yourself ready for the first meditation.

And now allow yourself to go back to the age of about eight. Know that you are fully protected as you go and that anything that might arise is only a memory. Nothing can hurt you now. You have already survived everything. Allow your mind to open and encompass everything up to the age of twelve. You don't need the detail unless you particularly want to bring it to mind. All you need to do is sweep it all together into a big bundle that you're then going to cleanse, heal and let go. You're not there, you're here and nothing can hurt you now.

Take your time.

Now with a beam of love from your heart, wrap your child self of that time firmly, comfortably and securely. Hold your child so that s/he knows s/he is safe. Now send a beam of light to cleanse and heal that time. Let the light shine in through and around it, cleansing and healing it forever.

If you're able, send forgiveness to the people, the time, the events of that time and release yourself and them from any negative connection, keeping only the good. Now, take your time. If you are able, rise to a higher spiritual level and see that the people of then were doing what they were doing because of their own pain and process of the time. Forgive them. Let them go. (If you can't, don't worry; go to the end of this part of the meditation.)

And now if you can, raise yourself to the highest level and see that they were in fact teaching you what you needed to know in this lifetime. They were a necessary part of your process as you were of theirs. Send them gratitude for having played an important part in your life, and let them go (again don't worry if you can't—you can always come back to this).

Now all is clean and clear. With love and compassion, take your child self back into your heart as s/he deserves. Wrap her/him with endless love. When you are ready, begin to return to the room. Feel your physical presence. Move your toes. Put your arms around your body. Love it. Enjoy your human self. And when you are ready, gently return to behind your eyes. Feel the attachment with the earth and, when you are ready, gently open your eyes.

Take your time. Have a drink of water. Stretch a little. Enter whatever you wish into your journal.

Meditation 2

Choose a time when you will not be disturbed for at least an hour. Take the phone off the hook and enter into a comfortable relaxed state by focusing on your breathing and letting go of anything negative, as you've learned to do.

Allow a wave of beautiful healing light to enter at the top of your head and flow down through you, filling every cell and every atom of every cell with wonderful healing light. Healing. Cleansing. Balancing. Every cell now bathed in light. Feel the refreshing touch of the light. Feel the cleansing. Feel yourself in harmony.

And now, take your focus down from behind your eyes through the center of your neck. Down through your throat chakra. Down through the center of your chest and your heart chakra and focus now on that area in your upper abdomen where your solar plexus lies. See it—a beautiful golden yellow ball of light, your own personal sun, shining out in all directions, filling you with warmth, filling you with light. Feel its warmth. Allow yourself to gaze on its brightness. See the sunshine entering into all of your tissues from this wonderful glowing ball of light.

Now as you warm to the light, feel simultaneously its gentleness and its power. Feel the power now flowing in and out of the glowing ball of light. Feel yourself becoming powerful. Feel yourself more capable than ever. Feel yourself strong. Feel yourself able to do new things. Feel yourself able to accomplish whatever you wish to do. Feel the power flowing into all areas of your body. Feel that your limbs are stronger than before. Feel the power surging through your body. Feel it in warm waves coursing through you. Know that you are capable of new strength, new power. Know that you will use this power for your own good and the good of others. In this moment, make a pledge that you will use whatever power the universe will give you for your own higher good and the higher good of all. Make a commitment that you will never abuse the power that is given to you now. Affirm that you are ready to receive the power of the universe and to use it wisely.

Enjoy the feelings now passing through you. Enjoy the warmth. Enjoy the power. Enjoy the strength. Take your time. Enjoy.

Ask that this power may now heal you. Heal old hurt or pain. Heal any old wounds. Heal you. Feel the power. Breathe it now to wherever you wish it to go. Flowing like the sun. Shafts of glowing light. Heal yourself now.

Stay for as long as you wish in this golden yellow glow. And, when you're ready, knowing that you will forever have whatever power you need so long as you use it for the higher good of all, start to return, leaving the sunlight shining there. Start your return. Bring your focus back to your solar plexus. Allow the rays of light to come back to the wheel of light that will always be shining there, but for now visualize a beautiful golden yellow flower over the chakra and let its petals close into a tight, tight bud. Let its head droop in sleep.

And gently now, bring your focus back up through the center of your chest, back up through your throat, back up till once again you are behind your eyes. Feel yourself present. Feel your physical body. Move your toes. Feel your attachment with the earth. Feel yourself well grounded. Hold your physical body and be aware that you belong here in your physical state. Be present and, when you are ready, very slowly and gently open your eyes.

Have a drink of water. Take your time and when you are ready, record whatever you wish in your journal.

SEVEN

The Heart Chakra:
Healing the Heart

∾

Love is a night bent down to be anointed,
A sky turned meadow, and the stars to fireflies.
Love triumphs.
The white and green of love beside a lake,
And the proud majesty of love in tower or balcony;
Love in a garden or in desert untrodden,
Love is our lord and master
We shall pass into the twilight;
Perchance to wake to the dawn of another world.
But love shall stay,
And his finger-marks shall not be erased.

—Kahlil Gibran

From the grounding of the root chakra, we moved to the sacral to embrace our sexuality and gain flexibility and strength. The solar plexus allowed us to combine our power and our will to open to our potential. Now we come to the heart, the pivotal point of our spiritual ascent, bridging the earthly and the divine as the chakras below it hold us securely in our human state while those above beckon us to the spiritual.

From its site in the middle of the chest, spinning at the speed of green light, the heart chakra radiates its powerful healing energy not only to the farthest point of our being, but to the whole universe. Here in this one chakra are the functions without which we cease to exist as human beings within a matter of minutes—our beating heart and our life-giving breath. Here also, love, compassion and touch reside, as the heart chakra demands that we reassess our relationship with ourselves and our profound connection with everything else in the universe.

Air, breath—the most basic of our needs—is the element of this chakra. In fact, so basic is breathing that we rarely think about it unless it is threatened. And yet it's one of the few physical functions that's automatic but which we're able to control readily by changing its depth, rate and rhythm. Autogenic training (see Glossary) shows that with practice we can learn to change most of the functions governed by the autonomic nervous system: for example, our heart rate, blood pressure, circulation or digestive processes that were previously considered automatic and so beyond our control. The link between breathing and emotion is marked. If we're anxious, frightened or angry, we tend to breathe more quickly and deeply (hyperventilate). When shocked, we sometimes feel as though our breathing stops. Just focusing gently on your breathing and simply counting your breaths can help bring down high blood pressure, settle a racing heart, calm you when anxious and restore equilibrium within a matter of minutes. A little time spent each day sitting quietly meditating on your breath will be richly rewarded by an improvement in your immune system.

Why not try a little conscious breathing right now? Just close your eyes and focus on your breath. Breathe in slowly to the count of six and, as you do so, visualize yourself breathing in peace and tranquillity. Then gently breathe out to the count of six, breathing out any toxins, any anxiety and tension. Now allow a little pause to the count of two. Again, breathe in to a count of six and let feelings of peace flow through you, and as you breathe out, let go of anything you don't need, seeing your whole self being cleansed. A little pause to the count of two. Again, another breath, this time to the count of eight, and allow everything nourishing to flow in on your breath. Hold it for a couple of seconds as you absorb all the goodness from it and then let the breath go and with it all that you no longer need. One more breath, again to the count of eight. This time breathe in light and let it flow to every part of you, cleansing, healing and balancing. As you breathe out, allow your whole body to relax. Just let go. Feel your weight on the earth. Then when you are ready, open your eyes again.

Feel better? It took just four breaths and only a couple of minutes to raise you into a totally different place. If you do that once an hour or so, or whenever you remember, you will be surprised at the enormous difference it will make both physically and psychologically.

Now, feeling refreshed, let's take a look at love!

Love and Relationship

The energy of the healthy heart chakra is what we call love. It almost defies definition despite being the most talked about, written about, sung about topic in the universe. Some cultures have several words for it but, whether we are referring to the feeling between lovers, parents and children, friends, siblings, our pets, or that fervent veneration of God, the energy has similarities and we call it love.

Love that enhances, enriches, makes beautiful, makes wise. Love that allows all to be forgiven, resolves conflict and heals sores. It's love that enables us to have the most profound connection and, finally, union with others. Love that opens doors and crosses continents.

Love at the heart chakra involves the relationship of all things throughout the whole universe, allowing us to rise to the highest level within ourselves and to have compassion for all living things. It gives us exquisite joy in togetherness, but also exquisite pain in sadness and grief. It transforms the commonplace into the sublime, and touches not only our own lives, but the life of everyone with whom we come into contact. Its charismatic power draws others to us and inspires them with confidence and hope as it enables them to open their own hearts also and to love just for the sake of loving, with openness and enthusiasm.

From here to the pinnacle of our spiritual ascent is love in one form or another. Love tempered with power, love softened with sweetness, love strengthened by protection. Love enhanced by understanding. Love toughened by wisdom. Love made never-ending by the spirit.

Love at the heart chakra draws together the human need for relationship that we encountered at the sacral chakra and also the understanding that we'll find at the crown (see Chapter 10) to enable us to love in a way that not only encompasses all beings but also all times, and all space and flows into every deed. This is the love that has been called "divine love."

Love and Healing

On page 12 I described the first flutters of my spirituality, which occurred when I was four or five. It took me some years to learn what was happening and to gain some control over it, though it can still happen spontaneously and catch me unaware even today.

Though sometimes I wasn't quick enough to catch it immediately as it began, I eventually felt able to trace it as a strong, palpable current began to flow. I used to think it started in the center of my chest, but as I focused on it I realized that it comes in through the top of my head and runs down through me until it kind of explodes in my chest and then shoots out in all directions. Within seconds it fills all of me and I can feel it move out into my aura until I know I am radiating love, like a torch. Long before I knew anything about chakras, I could sense places in and around me where the energy seemed almost to halt for a split second and change a little before it passed on. I found that I was standing in a bubble of it.

Now of course I know how to open my crown chakra to let love and light flow in, to add to it inner vision at my third eye, to welcome it down to my heart chakra and to focus it until it becomes almost like a laser passing out through my heart chakra or through my hands or feet with great power and force. Or I can let it be soft and diffuse it like a gentle cushion. I can open it to flood a room and calm very difficult situations or just hold people who are distressed within it while they deal with whatever they need to. I use it to help people heal themselves by empowering them to utilize their own energy in whatever way they need in order to be well.

It's one of the most useful tools I have and since it's pure, spiritual love, it makes it very easy for me to love without exception. So can you! I know that everyone is capable of feeling it once they've done the work to clear their chakras.

Accepting Yourself As You Are

So what do we need to achieve before we can truly love as the heart chakra demands? It's difficult to truly love if we can't accept ourselves as we are and be at peace. The sacral chakra helped us balance the masculine and feminine within us. Now we're confronted with the need to balance body, mind and spirit so we can begin to love both ourselves and others in a way that grants freedom and encourages and supports the spiritual growth of all.

Sometimes people struggle with the concept of accepting themselves, thinking that if we accept things as they are we're somehow selling out and not striving for progress. But in fact it allows for exactly the opposite.

Acceptance gives us a springboard for growth and development, a bit of solid ground to stand on even if it's a bit of ground we don't like very much. It's neither complacent nor arrogant. I don't think I'm perfect and needing no further change. But I need to be able to say (and believe!) that at this moment I am what I am and that's fine. That allows me to handle myself with compassion and the kind of indulgence I may have when watching a child struggle to learn.

Now at last the door is open to unconditional self-love, enabling me to embrace both the possibility and the reality of change. And it's only in unconditionally accepting where I am on my path right now that I can start to accept others unconditionally too. Loving is supporting another's growth, learning and spiritual unfolding. However, accepting and respecting other people doesn't mean I necessarily choose to have them in my life. Sometimes the most loving thing to do in a relationship is to accept that loving means leaving so that neither of us continues to be hurt by a situation that just doesn't work.

The same goes for acceptance of the way things are in society or on the planet. I need first of all to accept things as they are and flow love into the situation before I can decide what's the most loving way forward for me. Do I stay within the situation, or is my next move to leave it? Do I actively try to help change it? And if so, how can I do that lovingly and most effectively? What action would result in the most loving outcome all around?

In almost every case we can reframe things so there's a loving solution for all concerned, and that may include a decision to move myself and my life away since I don't really want my life to be infected by the way others choose to live theirs. There's a book by Gerald Jampolsky called *Love Is Letting Go of Fear*. The title just about sums it up. If we let go of the fear, we can learn to love in a much broader, more wholesome way.

Often people seem to see love as a limited commodity, like a cake to be cut. If I get a big slice, someone else gets a smaller one. There's a better way to visualize it. How about imagining love as a handful of balloons each filled with a special love for a particular person, individual, made to measure, a perfect fit. I can hold many, many balloons in my hand at once and everyone I love can have one. Not only that, but each unique and exquisite balloon can remain full, no matter how many balloons I'm holding. And if I'm not physically with someone, I can still be holding their balloon. I can gaze at it, relishing its beauty and think of that person, and the love flows between us as though we were together. Even if we never see each other or share time together again, their balloon can remain filled with all the things we shared, the mutual appreciation we've felt and the joy of the memory of the quality time we've had together. There's no need to be afraid that anyone else can ever have their share. And if I decide I want to let go of a balloon because the person it belongs to is no longer part of my life, with a loving thought I can let it float off to the heavens. No one gets less. Everyone gets enough. That's love.

Love and Jealousy

I often ask people what they mean when they say they love each other. Usually the responses include wanting to be together, finding each other appealing or attractive, feeling lost when apart, needing each other. But the most important part of love often seems to be absent.

That is the aspect of freedom, of wanting the other to be whole and healthy and all they can be, whether or not that includes us. The problem is that extra aspect of loving can be threatening, since it brings with it the possibility that the person we love may grow away from us and leave us behind. We may have to learn to be alone again. Often we respond to that fear by clinging, as though by doing so we could stop their process and hold them forever. But that need to hold and almost to possess isn't really love at all. It is dependence. And it's dependence, born of our own lack of confidence and self-esteem, that so often causes problems by allowing jealousy to develop. It robs love of its divine aspect and renders it commonplace, eventually destroying it altogether.

Our spiritual growth is the sole purpose of our sojourn on the planet and the journey continues without pause. Even if we take a breather and opt out of taking active control for a while, perhaps because we feel tired or just can't be bothered with the effort anymore, neither time nor our process stops. We're still making constant progress, constantly learning, constantly growing, passively absorbing life and its lessons.

If we try to remain the same and refrain from growing, to accommodate someone else's need for us to stay the same, the only long-term outcome is resentment, which kills whatever emotion there was. Real love never restricts us nor demands that we stop developing.

Letting Go with Love

Often when I talk about detachment, people seem to think I must mean attachment since, on the face of it, it seems to make more sense to be attached to what we love. But at the heart of real love is freedom. And freedom is about letting go. It's detachment that holds us together as we respect each other enough to have confidence that the other can live their life without us getting in the way and interfering with whatever process they need for their growth and development.

The healthy heart chakra allows us to remain detached and gives us a wonderful sense of unrestricted breathing, freedom and space, to say nothing of extra time to live our own life while still remaining supportive and truly loving of others.

So does unconditional loving exist? Yes it does. But I sometimes say to those I love that although I respect the fact that they may have to do what they do in a certain way, I don't have to like it. Unconditionally loving someone, and truly accepting them as they are, doesn't mean I have to either like or accept their behavior.

Loving you but not your behavior is often where the theory of unconditional loving comes unstuck. You and your behavior are not synonymous. Think of your behavior as a cloak that you wear for some specific purpose. Sometimes you get so used to wearing it that everyone, including you, thinks it is part of you. It isn't. Really you're underneath, just hidden from view for a while.

You can choose to take the cloak off or change it for a more attractive one. The responsibility for the cloak I choose to put on is mine and I can't expect that if I continue to hide behind an unpleasant one people will be loving enough to stay around. The same goes for you too. I have no right to try to change anyone (it would be a futile exercise in any case!). If I did I would be missing the very core of love—to give the other freedom to become all that they can be.

Their idea of being whole and healthy may not be the same as mine and who is to say who's right? Everyone needs to be allowed to find their own peace in their own way. So, I go on loving you unconditionally while not liking the behavior and preferring that you do it differently. But no matter how I may love you, if your behavior continues to be abhorrent to me, there may come a time when I'll continue to love you but choose not to have you in my life anymore.

Knowing When It's Time to Leave

Often people will get into a relationship feeling a karmic connection (see Glossary), that they've lived a life together in the past, and feel that this is the most amazingly wonderful, fairytale love that there ever was, only to find, a few months down the line, that they have little in common and need to part.

In days gone by, long engagements were designed to sort out such relationships from those that are based on stronger stuff and will survive.

As we get to know each other and then as we continue to grow, we become aware of areas of disagreement or conflict that may over time become so numerous that we become incompatible and the relationship is rendered untenable. Such incompatibility may then force separation, sometimes after only a brief period and sometimes after many years. If there has been a true connection at the heart chakra, love can remain, even though incompatibility dictates that there can never be togetherness again in this lifetime.

Being in internal harmony and balance is far more important to us in the long run than being in balance with other people, even those we love. Indeed, some people seem to spend their whole lives appearing to be out of balance with what the world thinks, but they're happy because they're being true to themselves.

If a relationship is so out of harmony that accommodating anything we disagree with or don't like takes us out of balance within ourselves, then we have to do some serious thinking about what we're still gaining from staying there. Sometimes, having accommodated and compromised for years, one small thing pushes our tolerance to the point where we're left without our inner integrity, and separation becomes inevitable. Tolerance, particularly in a relationship, is rather like a piece of elastic. We usually set out with a certain amount of it but when someone behaves in a way that's insulting or damaging to us, it will stretch, sometimes too far for our own good! How many times have you said, "I just wouldn't stand for that!" only to find that when it comes to the test, you do tolerate the behavior, forgive, but vow that you'll never accept a similar situation again.

When it does happen again, you increase your tolerance once more to accommodate it. You may do this several times, but as the tolerance elastic stretches and stretches you approach a point where there is very little give left in it. We may give verbal warnings to others that we can no longer cope with the situation, but even we don't listen to ourselves and of course our behavior is saying something else.

However, it happens once too often and suddenly our tolerance is gone. The elastic snaps back and we've passed the point of no return. Not only can we no longer tolerate the behavior, but our tolerance of it is far less than it was in the first place. Our mixed messages are over and we now have one foot out of the relationship.

Sometimes, even though the other person may make the changes we wanted and the relationship may trickle on for a while, it really ended at the point where the tolerance gave way. We may desperately want to make it right and keep it going, but deep down we know. Although we may put off the decision for a considerable time, eventually we have to leave.

The bond at the heart chakra which has been strong enough to hold us together through considerable trauma has frayed and snapped. What we have to deal with now is the pain of healing the place where the rupture occurred. The lesson is to set our boundaries realistically and lovingly in the first place and to try to keep them there. A normal part of the process of being in love is that from time to time we want exclusivity. Probably the best relationships are built upon the understanding that monogamy and mutual respect coexist. But this needs to be a gift that is freely given and not something that is exacted from the other under threat. The essential part of love is freedom—freedom to be, freedom to grow, freedom to become all that we can be and freedom to leave too if we must, without risking hatred or revenge.

Falling in Love

Falling in love, becoming infatuated and becoming dependent can all feel very much alike. Although it may feel like the real thing, some relationships are short-lived and pretty chaotic.

What makes us fall in love and what keeps us loving are two different things—a bit like the substance abuse we looked at in Chapter 4.

We looked at the masculine/feminine balance at the sacral chakra and at how we tend to look for someone, or be attracted to someone, who will balance our own makeup. There are of course other factors at play, including our personal experience, the relative strengths and weaknesses of our parents and what we've learned during our childhood. It has been said that girls marry their fathers and men marry their mothers. Sometimes, however, we look for someone exactly the opposite. Our fathers are our first male role model, and our mothers our first female role model. Much depends on whether we like them or not. Though sometimes even if we don't, and we look at our mother (or father) and say, "I'd never put up with that," we end up following the same track.

A man on a plane told me about himself and his brother and how they'd chosen different routes in life. They had a difficult and abusive father who drank heavily and beat their mother. One son, though drinking a bit too much, had nevertheless done quite well and was married with two grown children who were happily settled in their own lives. The other had been in a stream of trouble since adolescence, had been divorced twice and had very little but pain to show for his life. Someone had asked them separately why they thought they'd chosen such different lives. One had replied, "How could I have been any different when I had parents like mine?" The other had made exactly the same reply.

There's obviously much about both of these men that we don't know, but the point is we have freedom of choice. We have different life plans, different temperaments, different tolerance and different karmic baggage.

Falling in love and staying there is often the result of a long and ancient connection with a soul mate (see Glossary) with whom we've reincarnated in one form or another many times and who we know deeply on a spiritual level and with whom we have much in common. Dependence is something else again.

For two people to fall in love and for their relationship to proceed to healthy long-lasting loving, generally they both need to be quite independent and healthy in the first place. Have a look at the two people A and B in Figure 9a and see how they proceed as compared with the couple C and D in Figure 9b.

Here two healthy people with good individual boundaries with healthy heart and solar plexus chakras come together and are attracted to each other. They move toward each other but hold their boundaries intact as they begin to develop a friendship, feeling enriched and happy in each other's presence. Then comes the point when they fall in love (the

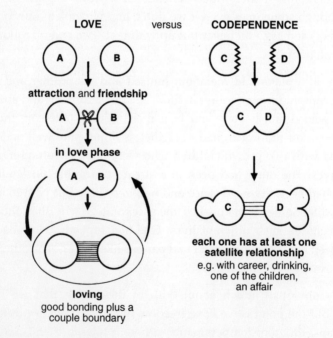

Figure 9: Love versus Codependence

time we talked about in Chapter 5). They suddenly let their boundaries fall and flood into each other, forming an amorphous blob in which one hardly knows where s/he ends and the other begins.

Do you remember that? Feeling like you were walking on air, doing things you usually wouldn't do, being up until all hours of the night, writing poetry, sending letters, making phone calls, telling friends and family inappropriate details, and so on. Been there? Done that? I have.

This phase can be quite exhausting, but since we're running on adrenaline with our chakras wide open we usually hardly register the fact that we're using much more energy than usual, getting very little sleep and often not eating very much either. But this can't last. There has to be a time of reckoning when we come to terms with our energy debt, and often it happens when she realizes for the twentieth time that he leaves his underpants on the floor for her to pick up, or he gets fed up with the top being off the toothpaste. Suddenly we wake up to the fact that this other person is in our space, and our boundary snaps back, leaving us very closely bonded to the other, but aware of what's ours and what's theirs psychologically and emotionally speaking.

Now a boundary that envelops them both and indicates to the world that they're a couple develops. They can be apart from each other (though they may not like it), secure in the knowledge that they love each other and have a deep bond that will hold them together.

There'll be wonderful times in this relationship when, perhaps during a holiday, a weekend away, or even just an evening together, they fall in love again with all that that means. Then they return to work on Monday morning feeling wonderful and within a few hours as they get on with the normal daily grind, they gently move back to the loving stage. This couple may alternate many times between being in love and loving in the course of their relationship, keeping it fresh and exciting.

Should they decide to no longer be together, though there'll be pain as they begin to dismantle the bonds, particularly at heart and solar plexus level, they may do so without acrimony. After an initial separation they may remain friends.

Now let's look at the second couple at 9b. Neither of them feels complete and they come together from a standpoint of need as they search for someone else to make them feel whole.

They're so eager to have someone to love and to be loved that they drop their boundaries very quickly, often bypassing the friendship phase, and become joined in that same amorphous mass. The problem is that because they felt so lost and less than whole before the relationship began, they're reluctant, and sometimes unable, to move apart when things start to go wrong.

It's difficult for them to communicate their true needs to each other since there's fear that in doing so they may lose each other. So, on all levels, they become stuck, locked into an unhealthy situation that allows for little if any movement or growth for either of them. Painful struggle between them may continue for a very long period since being apart means having to cope with being alone again and often they prefer to suffer the abusive situation.

This is the co-dependent relationship, each being dependent on the other to feel whole. Often the only way for them to develop a bit of freedom in the relationship is to take on another "satellite" relationship. This may be with another person (for example the woman may develop a very strong bond with one of her children) or with some activity (perhaps drinking, working too hard or having an affair).

The ending of such relationships is often peppered with acrimony, bitterness, sometimes violence and threats of, if not actual, revenge.

This reminds me of Michael, who came to me with a drinking problem and who gave a very elaborate account of why he got drunk, mainly blaming his wife with whom he obviously had a typical love/hate relationship. He stumbled through his history, which was blatantly a fantasy with poorly veiled lies about the level of his drinking and other addictive behaviors including sexual encounters with other women, for which he blamed his wife for being frigid.

He was capable of functioning creatively with some vision (his story was quite creative in itself), but he had so little sense of self and of his own boundaries that he manipulated others around him with a total lack of respect for theirs. He would hook others into his world by whatever means available and then he'd hold on tight, meeting any attempt the other might make to live their own life in their own way with a histrionic, aggressive display.

His wife, Margery, had been caught in this bind and was now attempting to get free. She was having therapy to deal with her pain as she witnessed the disintegration of what she described as a fairytale romance. She still exhibited her own dependence, however, and had another lover waiting in the wings since she couldn't face the possibility of being alone. Both needed to learn that they could function alone and without any of the crutches they had previously used, including each other.

Though each partner in the co-dependent relationship can eventually get well and become whole, sometimes in the process the relationship will fall apart. As Michael began to get well, one of the things that he had to deal with was that Margery had run out of tolerance for his behavior and needed to leave. Even though she had begged him to stop drinking, when it got to that stage, it was just too late.

Separation, Divorce and the Grief of Loss

Because of the bonds that develop between the heart chakras of any two people who open to each other in love, separation is never easy. The deeper the love they've felt for each other, the more exquisite the pain of the loss.

Similar pain can be experienced in other kinds of separation—for example the loss of a home or exile from one's country—as the heart bonds are suddenly wrenched apart. There's a meditation at the end of this chapter that will help if you find yourself in some grief.

Though the chakras are very rudimentary in the unborn child, the parents are already developing heart bonds with the expected baby. Should the pregnancy not reach full term, or the child is stillborn, the parents need to be given considerable help to heal the wounds of separation. This is something we used to ignore, though generally it's dealt with better now. Phyllis Krystal pioneered wonderful work on separation in her book, *Cutting the Ties That Bind* (Samuel Weiser, 1993).

Whether by choice (for example in divorce) or not, the heart bonds still have to be dismantled, severed and healed. Often much of the grieving is done before physical separation takes place, for example where there is advance warning of death. In couples who are parting, there's often spiritual and emotional separation by at least one partner long before they part.

Dysfunction at the Heart Chakra

Balance throughout the system is essential and, as this chakra more than any other lends itself to extremes, that's sometimes difficult to achieve.

The person who has a well-balanced heart can usually perceive the world optimistically as a kindly place overall, even when things are difficult, but with your heart blocked this becomes difficult. Negativity and pessimism can be overwhelming, obliterating the goodness there is.

As a society, we sometimes appear to have a heart chakra block: only bad news is reported and we seem to be eager to read all the sad, shocking and painful details of people's mistakes and misfortune.

Trauma or emotional pain around the age of twelve to fifteen or sixteen will have its effect on the developing heart chakra. Many people come along to see me feeling vulnerable and rejected, unable to feel loved or loving, their heart chakra clamped shut. Often they're critical and difficult to please, hold grudges and have difficulty with relationships. They often dislike some people, even feeling hatred and wanting revenge for perceived insults, while idolizing others who are seen as able to do no wrong. They see rejection everywhere and will often either withdraw or retaliate in pain, making it difficult for those around them to relax and be spontaneous. Their attitude will often deprive them of the closeness they so desperately want.

Those who've been involved in co-dependent relationships often have great problems with their heart chakra. Evelyn was one such case. She'd been living with the great love of her life for about seven years when she finally came along for some help. A tall, attractive, bright woman, she spoke articulately and was obviously perceptive and quite spiritual. She described her lover, Terry, as a wonderful man with whom she'd fallen in love almost at first sight. They'd had a stimulating, exciting relationship with great sex, lots of affection and had both been financially secure enough to travel and have whatever they wanted materially.

People had seen them as a golden couple and she was aware that others had envied their love. What she'd never shared with anyone, however, was what really went on from time to time in their relationship.

She had known from the beginning that Terry used drugs, though he said it was all part of the business world he moved in and wasn't a problem. Everyone did it and if he didn't he'd lose some of the contacts and leads that he usually made while "partying."

Although Evelyn didn't like it and had never been in a situation before where anyone used drugs, she said she thought it would change and had tried not to make an issue of it. Over time, however, she became aware that it was a problem. Money that she'd thought would be spent on their home or on holidays would disappear, and whenever he was confronted about this, Terry would become very defensive and angry. But what had distressed her more than anything was her own reaction. She remained deeply in love with him, she said, but she'd become so angry with the situation that she could no longer deal with it. She admitted with lots of tears and with downcast eyes that she'd become physically violent with Terry, and although he never retaliated, she couldn't live with the thought of what she'd become capable of. She knew that it couldn't go on like this. She no longer liked herself and sometimes now could hardly bear to look at him. She was afraid of what she might do someday because her tolerance was so minimal. She sobbed as she said that sometimes she was so full of rage she could kill him.

As a nurse, Evelyn was drawn to helping others partly because of her own family experiences. Her father had been a heavy drinker and she and her family had suffered greatly when he had died in an accident when Evelyn was fourteen. She was left with a mixture of love and anger that she'd never been able to sort out. She'd been stuck with her heart chakra wide open and Terry had walked straight in. She'd done all she could to love him better, had rescued him by telling lies for him, just as her mother used to do for her father.

She'd kept the truth from those who loved her. And now she'd lost her tolerance and had clamped her heart shut to protect herself from further hurt. She felt she'd lost part of herself that was very precious. At thirty-four, she wanted to start a family but knew it wouldn't be good to become pregnant in such circumstances. She was grieving for the dream of the relationship, the loss of herself and also of her childhood and her father.

The first thing was to teach her to open and close her heart chakra at will so that she could receive and give the good things but protect herself from further harm. There was grieving to do and practical issues to be sorted out. Where would she like to be and what would she really like to do if Terry's using continued? Could she cope with staying at their home? Was there a bolthole to go to if she needed to? How could she give Terry a direct and loving statement about her new way of treating the situation and follow through so as not to give him mixed messages? How could she set up a support system for herself, which would of course involve telling the truth to someone she could trust? And how could she get in touch again with that spiritual part of herself that she loved and felt she'd lost?

She was amazed to find that a very simple exercise of visualizing a beautiful green or pink flower over her heart chakra and gently watching it open and close immediately gave her some control over the amount of pain she felt.

She decided on a particular course of action for the next time Terry used drugs. She would make an assertive but not aggressive statement about her own needs and about what she was going to do. She would leave the house and try to stay away for a given time before she returned. In that time, she would try to nurture herself and be gentle with herself, say her affirmations and try not to send hateful vibes to Terry which would do neither of them any good.

In the meantime, she would tell him she was having some therapy and that she hoped he would too. Also, that she was going to make a decision as soon as she was able about what she wanted to do with their relationship.

Evelyn was surprised that once she changed her behavior, his changed almost immediately. He didn't stop using at once, and in the longer term he had to have some therapy. But, as Evelyn started to regain some of her self-respect, they were able to talk again and regain some of their trust and friendship. As she began to rebuild her life and see that she could live without him if she had to, the dynamics shifted. She moved out of co-dependence to a position where she could look to her own needs. Now the relationship at last became equal and they were able to move toward a real partnership, their marriage enriched by their individual growth.

Many people like Evelyn with dysfunction at the heart chakra are at the point where they dislike themselves as well as the situation/other person. They will exhibit self-denigration and self-loathing and often find it hard to empathize with others. In some, there may be difficulty in achieving emotional maturity and a tendency to deny responsibility.

A negative attitude pushes others away and fulfills the individuals' belief that they're unlovable. Since one of their great fears is of rejection, they'll often sabotage relationships so that they know where they are and have some control rather than waiting anxiously for the axe to fall. One of the hallmarks of the person who's stuck in negativity is to deflect any offer of help with a series of sentences beginning, "Yes, but . . ." eventually exasperating even the most gentle and attentive of caretakers. Badly needing tenderness, they're usually embarrassed by it, sometimes ridiculing others' finer emotions.

Often, though by no means always, those whose heart chakra has lost that ability to open and close at will are in some caring profession.

TOUCH AND COMPASSION

The sense of the heart chakra is touch—touch in its physical sense (tender strokes, loving hugs, massage) but also in a compassionate emotional or spiritual way. How much do you allow yourself to be touched? Do you allow compassion to enter into your life?

Perhaps you allow so much to touch you that you're rendered ineffectual by your pain, as you're dragged down by the suffering you witness. Being able to detach a little is more productive for everyone in the long run.

And are you in touch? In touch with the world around you? With the difficulties others are having? Perhaps they show their love for you in ways you just don't see because of preconceived ideas of how it should be. Why not look past what's being said and try to see how the other person is trying to get their message across to you. Maybe they just don't communicate as well as you. Are you hearing what they're not saying? Are you saying all you could? Are you being compassionate about where they are in their lives? Or are you being so understanding that you make excuses for them and allow yourself to be abused? Mainly, be compassionate with yourself. Allow yourself to touch and be touched in whatever way you can cope with now.

Desperate to help, everyone else's pain finally becomes too much of a burden to carry. Their worst nightmare is realized as they become burnt out, ineffectual and exhausted simply because they haven't learned the art of detachment. They are stuck with an open heart chakra that picks up and experiences everyone else's feelings.

Blocking at the heart causes our emotions to become distorted. If we're unable to detach and accept, we're unable to see the whole picture. There are many examples of how "love" has been distorted with tragic results. Some people passionately try to change one thing, but in their blinkered attachment and zealous defense of their cause they lose sight of the fact that they're creating another injustice and another set of victims further down the line.

Those who protect the rights of the unborn child for example by harming those who perform abortions, or those who fight for animal rights by harming the human beings who work in certain laboratories, have simply alienated many and harmed their own cause. If we come from the broader perspective of love and acceptance there's always a better and more powerful way—and that is to breathe love to wherever it is needed most.

The Exercises

Exercise 1

A healthy heart chakra leads to a positive outlook and an optimistic attitude that can change your life. First let's look at what happens when we're negative.

Let's say I have a negative thought, for example, "I'm unlikeable." I'll assume that no one likes me. Since I'm now prepared for people to dislike and reject me, I may not act in an open and friendly way. This negative behavior will prompt a less than friendly response and now I have negative feedback which only goes to confirm my negative belief that I am unlikeable. I'm set up for a whole new cycle of negative thoughts, assumptions, behavior and feedback which I keep on repeating until I find myself lonely and isolated. But actually I set the whole thing up myself without anybody else really doing anything. I set the stage, wrote all the scripts, played all the parts and got to the final curtain by myself!

Now let's turn the cycle around: I can open my heart and take a risk to have a positive attitude. Maybe I am likeable. If so, then others may like me and so I smile and—surprise, surprise!—people smile back. This positive response affirms that I am likeable. My self-confidence rises. Now I'm able to take more risks as my self-esteem grows and my world opens out, leading me to a happier state.

So, I'd like you to make a commitment to practice some positive thinking every day and to put it into action. Here are some affirmations to get you going, and though I'm not suggesting they'll cure all that ails you, they will have a profound effect on your heart chakra and on your mind since it believes every word you say. Remember that the best affirmations are the ones you make yourself, so play with them until you feel that they are just right for you.

- My heart is open to give and receive love and I am achieving perfect harmony and balance in my life.

- My first responsibility is to myself, to treat myself with love and compassion.

- My life is filled with possibility, wonder and delight. I only have to open my heart to receive.

- I flow love into every situation in the sure knowledge that love is flowing into my life.

Exercise 2

Write a letter to yourself as you might to your best friend, telling of your worries, your frustrations, your wishes, your goals and the things you're proud of and that please you. Say what's good in your life and what you would really like to change. Seal it and three or four days later sit in your safe place and read it carefully with compassion and understanding.

Now, from a very loving perspective, write a reply saying how you feel about what has been happening and making suggestions about what needs to be done. Perhaps you could make a list, but don't expect to do it all today. Where could you start? What one small change could you make today? There's always something. Now make a realistic time schedule for making changes.

For example:

- Starting today I can remember to treat myself as I would treat my best friend and every time I think or say something bad about myself I'll change it to something more appropriate and kind.

- Today I'll look in the phone book for an exercise class I can join.

- On Tuesday I'll buy myself some flowers when I do the shopping.

- I'll give myself a budget to spend on things that are important for my well-being and spiritual growth, for example some healing music, some candles, a crystal, some healing oil.

- On Friday I'll get out my old swimming certificate and put it where I can see it and feel proud of my accomplishment.

- Every day I'll massage my body with some perfumed lotion or oil after my bath or shower and book a professional massage when I can afford it.

- The next time my sister calls and says she and her family are coming for the weekend, I'll ask for time to think it over to decide whether that's convenient for me.

Exercise 3

Since I want my mind and spirit to be filled with good and beautiful things, I try to feed it a diet of good news, positive thoughts, healing music, pleasant memories, loving actions, sweet perfumes, gentle touches and uplifting sights.

I don't want it to be churning over disaster, murder and tragedy, so usually I don't read about those things or watch them on film or television. I know they exist and am not burying my head in the sand. I can send out love and healing to victims and perpetrators everywhere and also to those I know are struggling with the painful agendas they've set for themselves in this lifetime.

Is your mind being more troubled than it needs to be because of what you feed it? Is that helpful to you? Perhaps you could ask yourself if you'd be willing to put the equivalent in physical terms into your body. What do you think would happen to you if you fed it bad food, poisonous substances and unclean water? Take an overview of your life and see where your current negative beliefs come from. Do you still need them? Are they "old tapes" that have been playing in your head since you were a child? Do you want to re-record them with something more positive and appropriate?

Exercise 4

Make a list of five demonstrations of goodness you've been aware of today and add to it by sending out good thoughts with love and light to at least five people. See if you could make this a daily discipline. It would be so healing to your heart, and to the hearts of those you send it to.

A word of advice. If there is someone you would like to send something good to but you don't want to have contact with them—perhaps someone you have made a wise and conscious decision to separate from—it would be better for both of you not to re-establish heart bonds that you have worked to heal. Better to send them light rather than love. They'll still receive the peace and healing you send, but without your heart becoming involved again with theirs.

The Meditations

Meditation 1

As usual, go to your safe place and make sure you won't be disturbed for at least an hour. Have your crystal close by—a piece of rose quartz, green tourmaline or a piece of jewelry containing an emerald.

Rose quartz has been called the "love stone," so powerful is it to help us love ourselves and others. It's very healing to the heart if you're hurt and good at thawing out a heart that's been frozen in pain. Tourmaline comes in a variety of colors and green is both healing and protective, helping dispel negativity. Emerald signifies unconditional love and inspires kindness and prosperity as well as helping with insight. It's an old saying that we should only give jade to those we love since it carries so much love with it. If you have some jade this is a good time to use it. Before you begin, send some love back to wherever it came from.

If you want to burn some oils or incense, lavender or jasmine would be a good choice. If you have a flower or a plant, have that in your safe place too; otherwise have something green or pink around. Make sure the phone is off the hook.

You know the induction by heart now, so go through the usual routine to get relaxed and comfortable. Remember, anything that may arise is only a memory and nothing from the past can hurt you now. You have already survived.

This time you're going to go back to being between twelve and fifteen or sixteen and wrap together the events and the feelings of that time. Again, you don't need to bring to mind the details unless you wish to do so. Simply gather it all up in a bundle ready to heal. Take your time.

With a thought, allow light to shine into it, around it and through it. Let the light heal everything of that time and in particular the part of you that has remained stuck between the ages of twelve and sixteen. Let the light, and with it love, shine into every part of you and allow yourself to heal.

Now with a beam of love from your heart, wrap your young self firmly, comfortably, securely. Hold her/him so that s/he feels safe. The past is gone now.

If you are able, send forgiveness to the people and events of that time and release yourself from any connection. They have no connection with you nor you with them unless you want it. The past is the past and the past can be healed. Everything can be released now. As always, if you feel you're not ready to go on, stop here and return very gently to the room, grounding yourself before you open your eyes. If you are able, rise to a higher spiritual level and see that the people who did whatever they did then were acting within their own process and from their own pain and turmoil. Forgive them, let them go with compassion.

And now, if you can, rise to the highest spiritual level and see that these people were in fact teaching you whatever you needed to know in this lifetime in the only way you could learn it. They were a necessary part of your process as you were of theirs. Send them gratitude for having taught you and having played an important part in your life and let them go with compassion, with love and with gratitude. Take your time.

Now all is clear. With much love and compassion in your heart, breathe it into that young part of yourself and let there be peace and healing. Wrap yourself in endless love. When you are ready, gently prepare to return to the room. Feel your physical presence. Move your toes and fingers, put your arms around your body and love it. Enjoy your physical being. When you are ready, come back to behind your eyes and when you are truly here, feel the attachment with the earth. Feel yourself well grounded and gently open your eyes.

Take your time. Have a drink of water. Stretch a little. Then enter whatever you wish in your journal.

Have a break if you wish before going on to the final meditation.

Meditation 2

Close your eyes. Return once again to your safe place within yourself. Take your focus down to the level of your heart. Allow yourself to see a beautiful pink rosebud there. At the moment its petals are closed. See it in its as yet unformed beauty. Gently observe it and, when you are ready, breathe warmth and light into it and watch it begin to open. Softly, the petals start to move, slipping over each other, opening the bloom. Opening and opening to its full beauty. A wonderful, fully formed pink rose. Now it's at its peak, a spectacular bloom in all its glory. Though all of its stages of development were lovely, it is at its fullest blooming that it achieves perfection. The fully formed magnificent flower.

See this rose as the metaphor for your own blossoming. Now you are achieving your full bloom. Now you are at the peak of your blooming, you are, like the rose, fully opened, fully formed, stunning, beautiful, magnificent. This rose is your gift to yourself. You and your full flowering are a gift to the world. Hold the beauty. Hold the magnificence. You are the gift. Allow yourself to enjoy the feelings. Allow yourself to savor the moment. Allow yourself to embrace the magnificence of your maturity, your full flowering. Enjoy.

Now from the center of the rose allow a beam of love to go out to wherever you wish to send it—healing, cleansing, purest love. Notice that as you send it out you are healed by it also. Let it shine wherever it's needed most. Let it heal wherever it falls. Let this unconditional love heal the world. Let this unconditional love be your never-ending gift to the world.

Stay as long as you wish, and when you are ready, allow the beam of love to gently cease, though it will heal you forever. Allow yourself to hold on to the rose but enclose it in your heart now. Smile. Feel yourself healing. Enjoy. Take your time and when you're ready, gently bring your focus back to your physical body. Be aware of your weight on the floor. Allow yourself to be well grounded, in touch with the earth. Gently begin to stretch and be totally aware, returning your mind to the room. Make sure you're back to that place behind your eyes. Feel your physical body. Put your arms around it. Hold it, love it.

When you're ready, very gently open your eyes. Take your time. Just be.

Grief Meditation

Take yourself to your safe place and have some flowers and your crystal (rose quartz would be perfect) and, if you wish, a photograph or some object that reminds you of the person or thing you are grieving (for example a home you had to leave or a treasured item you lost, perhaps even the childhood you would have liked). Focus on your breathing and with your out-breath let go of anything negative through the soles of your feet and through your base chakra.

Spend a few moments being very gentle with yourself and allowing light to flood into you and be all around you. Bring to mind the person or thing you're grieving and allow yourself to feel the feelings that surround the loss. Remind yourself that you have to get on with your life and that though it may be painful to let go, you know you must do this in order to be free to continue your own growth.

Now gently focus on the object of your grief and imagine this person or thing in front of you. Give a message that you now need to heal yourself and that you're doing so with love for yourself and with love for them.

Allow beautiful white light to enter into the top of your head and let it fill you, entering into every cell and every atom of every cell until you are filled with light, radiant and healing. Note that it shines right to the palms of your hands and can shine out of them through the minor chakras there. Now, with a deep breath filled with love, let go of the beloved. Cup your hands around your heart and with that stream of healing light flowing from your palms heal the wounds left as the bonds were pulled apart.

If you have a partner or relative who is suffering the same loss, for example if you have lost a parent, had a child who died, or had a miscarriage or an abortion, or if you have a sibling who suffered the same loss and trauma during childhood, it's quite wonderful to do this together. Prepare yourselves well by talking about what you're grieving and by discussing what you're going to do. Read through the meditation together, then let yourselves fill with light, and each cup the heart of the other simultaneously. Allow the love to flow between you as you heal yourselves and each other. Let go of what was lost and spend a little time talking about the experience both of the loss and of the healing experience you have just shared. End with some form of supportive physical contact such as a hug or holding each other's hands and take your time before you part to get on with your day. Choose a day when you can spend time together without interruption and without the fear of guests arriving. It is a good idea to involve other children or the family if there has been a death in the family.

EIGHT

The Throat Chakra: Speaking Our Truth

Let there be many windows in your soul,
That all the glory of the Universe may beautify it.
Not the narrow pane of one poor creed can catch the radiant rays
That shine from countless sources.
Tear away the blinds of superstition;
Let the light pour through fair windows,
Broad as truth itself
And high as heaven.
Tune your ear to all the worldless music of the stars
And to the voice of nature,
And your heart shall turn to truth and goodness as the plant
turns to the sun.
A thousand unseen hands reach down to help you to their
peace-crowned heights,
And all the forces of the firmament shall fortify your strength.
Be not afraid to thrust aside half truths and grasp the whole.
—*Ralph Waldo Trine*

We have ascended from our basic instincts of survival at our root chakra through the sacral with its accent on our sexuality and capacity to reach out to others. At the solar plexus we explored our power and finally came to unconditional love at the heart chakra. Now we burst into sound and communication as the fifth chakra, the throat, enables us to give voice. It brings together the emotions and instincts of the lower chakras and the vision, thought, knowledge and understanding of those above it. With a developed throat chakra, we can discover the gifts of better communication, creativity, integrity, clairaudience (see Glossary) and channeling.

The throat chakra bridges the feeling self and the intellectual self and also encompasses such things as wit and the ability to improvise, and these will be enhanced by its development. There's a lovely lightness as the throat chakra opens. You become less likely to take yourself seriously, more spontaneous and willing to play, to be childlike and "give it a try" while being able to snap into your power and command attention and leadership in an instant when necessary. You may seem almost like two different people as you switch with ease to the behavior appropriate for any given situation. It is the throat that allows us to express verbally what so far we have only learned to feel. This verbal expression lets us share who we are with the outside world and lifts us above and beyond other species. As we open our throat chakra and put our original unique expression into sound, we simultaneously take into our own world all those who hear us.

Sadly, we often speak carelessly and without due thought. However, as we recognize the responsibility of the spoken word, we learn to choose our words more carefully since, once released into the ether (see end of chapter), they can never be retrieved.

Improve Your Communication

The throat chakra moves us to communicate in speech. The spoken word is so important that it forms the opening statement of St. John's Gospel: "In the beginning was the Word." It is as though we as a species began with sound and language. Here at the throat we communicate as only human beings can, from a whisper to a shout, from a song to a scream.

But communication is not only about the word, be it spoken, written or broadcast. The loop of communication is completed by hearing and listening. Whether it is the clicks and whistles of dolphins, the chatter of children's voices, or the faintest change in a baby's breathing, the human ear is attuned to sound, albeit of a limited range compared with other animals.

Our understanding is further enhanced by non-verbal communication. We communicate internally, listening to our body and the signals it constantly gives us, listening to our soul as it gently guides us and listening to the universe and to the higher wisdom that's there like a constant backdrop. Like the sound of the cicadas in the trees on a tropical night, we become so used to it that often we no longer hear it. We need to stop and listen in order to hear its beauty and appreciate its full impact on our lives.

Without communication, thoughts and ideas remain solitary unexpressed intangibles and, apart from expanding the mind of the thinker, have little use. Communication grasps them, gives them body, shapes them and makes them real. Their energy is released into the world as we share what we know, gathering consciousness around our unique thoughts and allowing others to add their energy. It's like rolling out a bale of fabulous silk and allowing others to wonder at its beauty, to touch it and share the magic.

I have been known to say that all relationship problems come down to poor communication, and I don't just mean loving relationships— I mean those with colleagues and pretty much anyone and everyone we meet. And though that may be a sweeping statement, it's not far from the truth. If communication can begin with a smile, continue with love and civility, be leavened with a little humor when appropriate and enhanced with empathy and compassion, we can hardly fail.

Finding Our Voice

Our voice is a great gift. My closest friend has a wonderful voice that was surely brought from another time, so rich is its tone and so strong and emotive its quality. But sadly she uses it rarely, partly due to shyness.

We talked earlier about using what gifts and skills we have and building on them. I'm not suggesting that she should become a professional singer. She has other talents she can market for the good of all. But if we receive a beautiful present from a friend, we show appreciation, use the gift or put it on show so others can also admire it. Why not then with God-given gifts? Should we be falsely modest and pretend we don't have them? Or be rightfully pleased and willing to share? Whatever we have been given is to share with others in whatever way we can.

Opening our throats to sing ennobles us. But the best thing about it is it clears our throat chakra and therefore shifts blocks of communication, creativity and higher gifts. So if you can sing, fine. But even if you feel you can't, you can chant or learn a mantra (see Glossary) to repeat in a rhythmical way that will similarly open up your throat and make considerable changes in your life (see exercises, page 176).

Whatever you do, you could perhaps make it a rule that you always give gratitude with your voice. Though inner thanksgiving is fine, and there are times when a silent prayer is proper, you can open your throat and express gratitude at any time.

I'm sure that anyone who stays with me for the first time has a little chuckle in the mornings as I emerge from the bedroom and address everything along the way. First I say good morning to the morning, then to the sky, and bit by bit wander around the house greeting everything and saying good morning to it. I thank it for being there and performing whatever function it performs in my life. Sound crazy? Well, maybe, but voicing my gratitude sets up a loving vibration in my home.

It really pleases me when people tell me my home feels loving and peaceful. Partly it's that way because I do healing there, but also because I set up loving sound waves by talking, chanting, singing, clapping my hands and generally joyfully moving the energy. I also create wonderful sound with music, bells, wind-chimes, a gong and singing bowls and these please my ear, clear my throat chakra and set up a sparkling energy that lifts my mood and that of everyone who comes there.

Do you ever tell stories? Did you like to have a parent tell you stories when you were little? One of my friends and colleagues is a Jewish storyteller. He tells ancient stories that have been part of his culture for centuries, handed down by mouth rather than in a written form. On my fiftieth birthday I invited him with lots of other friends to celebrate my life with me and I asked him toward the end of the evening to tell us stories. What happened was quite magical. We put out all the lights and had only candles. As he began, the whole atmosphere changed. Everyone's energy shifted and we became mesmerized by his voice and the stories he was telling. Every now and then I dragged myself out of the almost hypnotic trance to watch what was happening. It really didn't have anything to do with the story, it was how we concentrated on his beautiful voice. All of our throat chakras were open and the love flowing between us was magnetic. The healing that took place that night was magical, such is the power of opening to our creativity, to communication and to love.

The Power of Being True to Yourself

The Sanskrit name for this chakra is *Visuddha*, which means pure. The healthy, evolved throat chakra moves us to refine the quality and purity of our communication. It behooves us to pull together our experience, power, will and love and to have the courage to put out into the world the truth as we know it. Truth which is not simply a collection of static facts, but a living, developing, dynamic process.

Truth is unique for each of us, tempered by our experience and growth. The facts are of course important, but the truth of the throat chakra is much more than this. It has integrity, depth and power and is a synthesis of all that we've learned so far on our journey. It is enriched by the intuition, wisdom, clarity and understanding of the higher chakras as we now express them to the world.

Our truth, then, contains our vision, our dreams, our hopes, our knowings, the results of the exploration of our thoughts and the deliberation of our hearts and minds. It is our highest integrity, and may differ from that of anyone else. Acting in line with our integrity may prompt us to have different standards or attitudes to anyone else's, and that's okay. For, once we know our own truth, we threaten our integrity if we ever cross the internal boundaries of conduct that that truth demands. Behaving in a manner discordant with our truth costs us in terms of regret, sorrow, loss, shame and a sense of personal grief that we didn't live up to our inner wisdom.

When we speak from an evolved throat chakra, we're generally heard, since not only does the message have the ring of genuineness, but the words are spoken with power, grace and clarity born of the higher chakras.

So the throat chakra calls us to get in step with our truth and have the courage to stand by it whatever the opinions of others. But we must remember to update the truth. What was my truth a few years ago, or even yesterday, or five minutes ago, may cease to be my truth now in the light of new experience, new facts and a new emotional state. The throat chakra requires me to have the courage to renew the truth and if necessary admit that however passionately I held a certain view a while ago, I now hold another.

This ability also gives me the compassion and understanding to accept that since we're all at different points in our evolution, we're at different points in the development of our understanding of the universal truth. So, differences of opinion and passionately held views can be supported and accommodated when seen as a product of time and process. They're merely snapshots in a continuing film.

As long as we responsibly share our own truth and are willing to hear that of other people, then there is ongoing evolution throughout the universe. This prompts us to hold the truth lightly and with flexibility, being willing to look at new facts and concepts in order to incorporate them into our lives, as you're doing with this book.

The throat chakra challenges us to have the courage and responsibility to stand up and say what we know to be the truth, to admit when we're wrong, to change our minds and to keep our truth alive and forever updated as new information arises. This last point is well illustrated by the following apocryphal story. A great general summoned his war cabinet in the morning and gave them his plan of campaign. They left and gave orders to the troops. At lunchtime he summoned them again and told them to ignore the plan of the morning and gave them new tactics. Again they left and put the new plan into action. At sunset, he called them back once more to his war office. He rescinded the instructions of lunchtime and presented them with yet another strategy. One of the generals complained that they were beginning to look foolish, having changed plans now three times in a day. The great general looked at him with compassion. "Would you like me to make this evening's plan on the basis of this morning's information, or would you prefer me to have the courage to do what is right, now that I am better informed, even if that makes me look foolish?" he said. They went on to win the war.

Finding Your Vocation

While the throat chakra at the front deals with general communication, the portion at the back of the neck focuses on getting our personal unique message out to the world. Our best opportunity to do this is via career and vocation.

Part of the work at the throat chakra is to define what we really want—where our heart is really leading us—and to have the courage to follow it. Already we've learned from the pleasure/pain principle of the sacral chakra that the universe will lead us by rewarding us with free and easy forward motion when we're on the right track and by gently putting obstacles in our way if we're not. All we need to do now is build on this and refine it so that we follow the right path.

There was a time when my life's work was to be a mother and look after my children. Then there came a time when I was a full-time doctor and healer. Now I'm continuing on my path which has led me to spend more time teaching, writing and channeling healing. I know that I have not yet reached my full potential and am dedicating my life to love, to peace, to healing, to teaching and to my continued spiritual growth and that of others.

Discover Your Creativity

As with every rung of the rainbow ladder, we use all that we've learned in previous chapters and incorporate it into our greater level of understanding. In this respect, there's a special link between the sacral and the throat chakra. The ideas that began to emerge at the lower level are now primed with the creativity of the fifth chakra and all things become possible.

So often I hear people say, "But I'm not creative." How sadly conditioned we are. Who told us that? Teachers who failed to put our drawings on the wall? Who didn't pick us to play Cleopatra in the school production?

We are all creative beings. As yet, some of us haven't unearthed that part of ourselves, but often that's because the throat chakra, which deals with creativity, doesn't really start to evolve until the age of sixteen. For many, that's just past the time when they're being daily stimulated and encouraged to develop, if indeed they ever were. The sad result is that some people never do enjoy this God-given inner resource and go on believing that they're less than others. I'm not saying we're all equally creative. We've all come to this life with unique gifts. I may be able to play a simple tune on the piano, but I know I wasn't born in this lifetime to be a great concert pianist. But I do have creative gifts to share and so do you. I'd have been one of the ones who would have said some years ago that I wasn't creative. But in the words of the song, "If they could see me now . . ."

Whatever we love doing shows us where our creativity lies. I run a workshop called "Doing what you love and loving what you do," which encourages participants to look at what gives them a kick and the skills they have. They can then build on those to develop a really prosperous lifestyle that's creative, is in line with their integrity, gives them joy, uses their energy in a positive way and earns them a good living. The payoff for the rest of the world is that in addition to being useful and effective they are radiating happiness and love around them because they are enjoying what they do. That's being creative.

Living According to Your Integrity

Living according to our integrity forms a major part of the work here at the throat chakra.

Just as my truth is a very personal issue, so is my integrity. It is a function of my truth and I have to act within it and incorporate its standards of conduct, which are dictated by both my understanding and my conditioning. The latter is largely a result of some of those invariables I chose when I decided to reincarnate this time. The fact that I was born to my wonderful parents in a little village in the northeast of England and had a very simple upbringing with country values, that I am a woman in the 20th century, is very important to the development of my integrity. It would have been different had I been born in a village in Ethiopia thirty years later or a palace in India a couple of centuries ago. Those invariables, my conditioning and my spiritual development, have shaped my integrity. It is at my throat chakra that I must have the courage to follow it in word and deed.

For instance, my integrity wouldn't allow me to spoil the environment by dropping a piece of litter without feeling shame but it would allow me from time to time to ignore a manmade edict that appears to have little relevance to my life. I have no doubt that if my children were dying of malnutrition my values would be different. I'm not suggesting here that it's okay to ignore laws and rules. However, I do think major progress occurs when, from the point of our integrity, we challenge what we perceive to be wrong, restrictive or unnecessary. Another one of those big throat chakra issues up there with truth and integrity is morality. It's another issue that's highly personal, variable and constantly developing according to our circumstances.

There used to be a television show that challenged participants to look at their morals by revealing only a little of a story at a time and asking what would be the best way forward. Usually people began by feeling one course of action to be morally right, only to find that, once they knew all the facts, they would have behaved in a totally different way. Though their high standards of integrity and morality had not changed, the circumstances that were presented caused them to make different judgments.

If I look back on my life I sometimes cringe at what I did, although I felt that my actions were acceptable for one reason or another at the time. Similarly, I have sometimes looked back and thought what I missed by having the values and morality I had. But I have to accept that that was where I was then. What was in line with my morality then, and what I felt to be just, isn't necessarily in line with my current understanding. I need to let go with love and forgiveness for myself and those around me at that time, accepting that it was an essential part of my process and theirs. The current development of my throat chakra (and all my others too) won't allow me to do some of those things now without a sense of guilt, but it will allow me to do others with impunity that I might not have contemplated five or ten years ago, or even yesterday.

Clairaudience, Channeling and Telepathy

The higher we move up the spiritual ladder, the more gifts we find. Some of the most wonderful bestowals of the developed throat chakra are clairaudience, channeling and telepathy.

Clairaudience is the gift of inner hearing, which is somewhat different to hearing with our physical ears. Even those who are deaf can develop clairaudience. I personally perceive it more as a knowing that appears to come from nowhere but which I "hear" with my mind.

Channeling is a phenomenon that has been around for centuries, though its quality has changed over the last few years. It enables us to open up channels to communicate with higher masters and to bring down, in language we understand, wisdom and teaching. This information has enhanced our knowledge about subjects as varied as "death," the universe itself, astrophysics and the essence of life. There are wonderful explicit teachings from such discarnate beings as Seth, Gildas and Orin to name but a few (see Bibliography).

ETHER

The element of the throat chakra is the ether, that unifying field from which everything arises and in which, like the ocean, everything swims. All particles, all matter, all things physical arise from this field, this matrix. But not only do they arise from it, they're part of it and they comprise it. Molecules that have been in existence since time began, that have been recycled, re-formed, changed and used in various chemical reactions, remain part of it. Though in places there may appear to be emptiness, this is just a place of sparse population of molecules, where little appears to be floating. There is no such thing as space. No such thing as separation between us. Everything holds some kind of connection, however infinitesimal, to everything else by means of the matrix, the ether.

In Chapter 7 I described how everything we do has a consequence. Here we refine that concept. Since we're all united and moving together in the universal matrix, if I make a loving gesture it will move all in its path, affect everything and eventually return to affect me lovingly also. The concept holds true if I do something that is not of pure intent. It will surely rebound, however long it takes.

Because mediumship that taps into the astral plane has had such a high profile, channeling that taps in at a totally different and higher level has often received critical press. True channeling, which is direct and precise, requires an open and unconditionally loving heart and a developed brow chakra and crown as well as an evolved throat chakra. As I have said earlier, usually those who are blessed with great powers are quite humble (not falsely modest) to have been chosen to have them. Beware those who flaunt their power, as such pride comes from the ego rather than the spirit.

A similar gift is that of telepathy, and we're all capable of this skill to some extent, especially with people we love or are particularly in tune with. Most mothers can tune in to their children and can feel when something's wrong even from a great distance. Lovers will know exactly what the other is thinking or is about to say (unfortunately they often lose this ability later when other forms of poor communication set in). Most of us will have been aware of the phenomenon of intending to phone someone when they phone you. Telepathy is in many ways an enhancing of these commonplace and often underestimated skills and is made possible by an evolved throat chakra. There isn't really any space between us. In the final analysis we're all joined in spirit. So if I send a mind message out into the ether the person I send it to will eventually pick it up.

Let's say I send out a loving thought to my son. The loving vibration of my thought goes off into the ether and homes in on its target: he will pick it up even perhaps on a level of which he's not consciously aware. To some extent it doesn't matter if he never realizes that the love comes from me; his life will be enhanced by it anyway. So I can change things dramatically by sending out loving messages. Similarly I could do a lot of damage by sending out hateful ones. But since everything will come back to me, I really need to be careful that all that I consciously, and unconsciously, send is loving and for the higher good of the person concerned.

In Chapter 7, when I discussed sending out forgiveness, I suggested sending light rather than love in some cases. That's very important if you don't want to get your heart chakra involved with someone from whom you wish to be separate even though you want to send them good things.

Telepathy is merely an extension, a sharpening, of this phenomenon. It's about being more aware of the messages that are being sent out as thought forms and being able to read them almost at will. Like all other spiritual skills it's open to abuse so be careful and don't invade people if you find that you're capable of telepathy. I'm also very wary of people who use spiritual gifts as party games and I avoid those who ask me to do so. It's inevitable that some people are fascinated by the unusual, but do try not to be drawn into that. Our gifts are to use in the way they were intended and I believe that, like any other gift, if we abuse telepathy we don't deserve to have it and will possibly lose it.

Dysfunction at the Throat Chakra

The throat chakra rotates at the speed of clear, bright blue light as it bathes the neck and all its organs—the throat itself, vocal cords, the thyroid and parathyroid glands and also the mouth, the trachea and esophagus, the ears, the cervical spine and the carotid plexus.

A blocked or sluggish throat chakra will often manifest physically in recurrent sore throats, colds, swollen glands, neck pain and dental problems. There may be symptoms of hypo- or hyperthyroidism. The former presents with lethargy, weight gain, low mood, coarsening of skin and hair and the latter with weight loss, anxiety, poor sleep and increased energy accompanied by jitteriness. (See Appendix A dealing with endocrinology.)

Melvin came to see me feeling angry and depressed. A very bright man in his thirties, he felt disillusioned with life. He said that wherever he went he found that people were initially pleasant and helpful, but that after a while they were not really interested in anyone but themselves. He'd moved around quite a bit and several times he'd thought that he'd found the right career, the right environment, the right girlfriend, but it always ended badly. Bit by bit, he was losing hope that there was anyone who had any integrity or even common sense. He seemed totally unaware of his arrogance and he went on to lecture me about the stupidity and insensitivity he was confronted with on a daily basis.

He talked clearly, with a lot of authority and a lot of words. I could imagine that first impressions would lead people to be attracted to his bright mind and his passion for his chosen topic. I could also imagine that after a while they'd become bored with the fact that he talked at rather than to them and ignored others' points of view.

Despite his highly articulate delivery, his colorful use of language and his enthusiasm for his subject, Melvin was lacking some of the essentials of good communication. He seemed unable to listen attentively, was thoughtless and had difficulty in accepting social cues about allowing the other person to speak. Not only did he miss much of what he could learn because he felt he already knew it all, but he gave the impression that no one was such an authority as himself. This undermined the esteem of most of those he came into contact with. I had no doubt that his colleagues would see him as rather bumptious and offensive as he challenged every light-hearted comment as being frivolous and accused others of lacking depth simply because they took themselves less seriously. To Melvin, life was a very serious business of black and white but no gray.

He demonstrated so well his throat chakra problem as he confused wordiness with communication. He took himself and the world very seriously and like so many others with a block at this chakra, was on some kind of crusade. Sadly, he and those like him do it little good because they alienate those around them by the ponderous nature of their attack.

Often they will be popular in the short term but finally they will alienate others and end up either feeling misunderstood or believe that they are surrounded by morons. However, they fail to recognize the golden rule that if you repeatedly end up feeling misunderstood, then you're the common denominator. It's probably your communication and lack of understanding that needs to be addressed. Blocked throat chakras lead to blocked creativity, which often means an endless, restless search for the right place in life. Small wonder that Melvin was running out of careers, places and girlfriends.

When we're on our path it's exactly that—a path. We're constantly moving along, climbing the next hill, changing things a little, adding and building on what we already have to get to where we're supposed to be. Our throat chakra is essential to this process. However, as with all the chakras, it doesn't exist or work in isolation and needs the vision of the sixth chakra, the love of the fourth, the power, will and potential of the third and the ideas and opinions of the second to fully blossom and lead us to our goal.

The Exercises

The crystals that are particularly useful for the throat chakra are turquoise and lapis lazuli. Apart from being a powerful protector, turquoise

AFFIRMATIONS

We've used affirmations throughout this book, and of course we've been using the power of the throat chakra to make them work for us. The power of the word as a creative tool can't be underestimated, especially if it is embellished with vision. The process of creating our world by affirmation can be likened to the process of creating anything else.

Let us say we have a beautiful chair. How did it come to be there? Well, someone, somewhere had a mental picture of what they could create. Then, they made a blueprint, a drawing or a verbal description of the vision. Next there may have been some refining of the blueprint, until it felt just right. Finally, the building process and, at last, the chair comes into existence.

Affirmations help us shape our world and change our lives in the same way. First we need to have the vision. What do you really want to create? We'll be looking more at that in the next chapter. But so often I ask people what they want and they don't know. No wonder they haven't created it yet. Remember what we said at the beginning of this book: Healing is an active process. You have to do it. There are those who will help guide you, but you and only you can heal your life. So what do you really want? Once you know, you can start to create it by the same process as that which created the chair. Affirmations are the drawing or the blueprint. You can actually make a drawing if you like—it's called a treasure map. Or you can make a collage and put it somewhere where you see it regularly so that you can keep focused on what you're creating. However, the fine-tuning and adjustment until it feels really right is a very important part of the process. Fortunately, this is simple to do with affirmations because you can change everything with a single word.

enhances communication, creative expression and emotional balance. Lapis lazuli strengthens the thyroid and also augments psychic abilities while inspiring greater creative expression and improving vitality. Silver is renowned for improving speech and strengthening faith in your higher self, so if you have some silver jewelry with any of these stones it would be good to wear them.

Suitable aromatherapy oils are lavender or hyacinth, which tend to be gently soothing, or patchouli or white musk, which will stimulate creativity.

Exercise 1

This exercise helps you clear your space with sound. Not only does pleasing sound nurture your sense of hearing and improve your creativity, it also enhances all your communication skills by clearing your throat chakra.

Pleasing sound for me includes the human voice, birdsong, music, bells, wind-chimes, the sound of the wind, thunder, running water, rain and much more. I find noise and discordant sound offensive and damaging to my throat chakra and when I am subjected to it, it takes me a while to settle down to being creative again.

Pleasing, harmonious sound is useful for changing the vibrations in the space you occupy and you might like to experiment with opening your windows and hanging wind-chimes where you can hear them, playing mood-changing music (see the next exercise) or investing in one or two recordings of natural sound such as rainfall or waves crashing on the beach. You can create your own sound of course by singing, clapping your hands, chanting, beating a drum, using a singing bowl. Whatever you choose, I think you'll be surprised at the difference it makes to the energy in your space and indeed your own personal energy. Try it!

Exercise 2

Music is the most mind-altering substance known to man, and it's legal! There are pieces of music that are right for particular chakras and I'm sure you will find what feels just right for you. It may be an earthy grounding piece for the root chakra, a flowing piece that tunes in to the water element of the sacral, a powerful stirring epic for the solar plexus or a gentle loving one for the heart chakra.

All of them are perceived at the throat chakra. Music is a very personal thing and our tastes change according to our development. But music for healing may be quite different from the music you want to play in your car or dance around to in your living room. If you want music to get lost in, to heal your chakras and to lift yourself into a different place, perhaps you'd like to try some of my favorites, but please do also find your own.

The piece of music I use to stir and lift the energy and do powerful healing, especially where the release of anger is concerned, is the soundtrack of *The Last of the Mohicans* (1992 version), especially the first track. It has an amazing quality and can move mountains as far as achieving catharsis (see Glossary) is concerned. Remember that catharsis is at its most beneficial when there is healing of the raw space left after the emotion has been expressed. So if you're on your own and you experience catharsis, follow it by something very soothing. For me the sound of pan pipes tunes in to my root chakra, as do drums.

For the second chakra you might like to try a recording of waves on the beach, rain falling or a brook. But there's also wonderful classical music that flows and will touch this chakra beautifully. I love Grieg and Chopin. Go and listen to some in your local music shop. The solar plexus responds to powerful, emotional music. A great mover for me is Rachmaninov's fifth piano concerto, written when he was himself coming out of a depression. Its minor chords are amazing in their ability to shift my emotions.

The soundtrack of *Out of Africa* (MCA Records, 1986) moves my heart, as do some of the beautiful piano pieces by David Lanz. There's so much romantic music both classical and modern that you'll be spoiled for choice. For the throat chakra you might like to try some vocal music. I like Gregorian chant and one of my favorites is *Canticles of Ecstasy* by Hildegard von Bingen (Deutsche Harmonia Mundi, BMG music, 1994).

For the brow, Terry Oldfield's music is lovely. There's quite a lot to choose from. However one of my favorites is *Music for Healing* (Stephen Rhodes, New World Music). For the crown the best music is silence! Nonetheless, I know some people who like natural sounds such as birdsong for this chakra. If you do want music, then *Return of the Angels* (Philip Chapman, New World Company) would suit.

FOR YOUR THROAT CHAKRA

Take some time for yourself, take the phone off the hook and settle comfortably in your safe place. Have your music ready so you can switch it on easily without moving around too much. For this exercise either sit or lie, whichever you prefer. Close your eyes. Take a few deep breaths, imagine a beautiful sky-blue flower at your throat and watch its petals open. Switch on your music and just allow the sound to take you wherever you need to go. You needn't actively listen unless you want to. Just be in the sound. Let it flow into you through your open throat chakra. Be part of it. Feel the power of it.

Allow the music to completely finish before you move. Now, take your notebook or journal and just allow whatever is in your mind to empty itself onto the page. Don't worry about the grammar, about it making sense, about spelling or anything else. Just let your hand keep moving and pour out whatever you have to communicate. Let it flow. Try not to think. Just let it appear on the page. If you feel it would be easier for you to speak than write, then have some recording device you can use. Afterward make sure to date it so you can keep it and look back on it.

Exercise 3: Chanting, Mantra and Sounding Your Note

Chanting is the art of saying or singing words or sounds repeatedly as part of sacred practice. It can be very effective for inducing changed states, enhancing awareness and focusing concentration as an aid to meditation.

There are some ancient chants and invocations you could use, or you can make your own using whatever words or sounds you wish. It can be very powerful to simply chant your own name, quietly at first and then altering the tone, power and texture of your voice, noticing what a difference that makes. You may find that you have a flood of self-love and self-esteem when you do this simple but powerful exercise. For me the word Om is all I need and I use it either as a chant, a mantra or to sound my note. The last is a practice that always precipitates initial amusement and / or embarrassment at workshops until its effect is appreciated. As you'll see from the instructions below, you can sound your note using any word or sound, and you can do it anywhere. This practice will also clear your space and shift the energy.

So, here's how. Close your eyes, focus on any of your chakras for a few moments, then fill your lungs with air and allow your throat to open and let yourself sing out whatever note feels comfortable. You can then play with singing it with gentleness and sweetness or with power and force. The energy both within your body and within the space around you will change completely as you set up a different vibration with the sound waves you're creating.

Now choose a different chakra. You'll find that the note you now sound will probably be different even without you thinking about it. This exercise is particularly good for singers or those who wish to use their voice professionally, for example for public speaking. Now, close your eyes. Focus on each of your chakras separately in turn without making a sound. Then focus on drawing the energy of the lower chakras up to your throat and the upper ones down to your throat. Now with the power of them all at once, open your throat and sound the note of your soul. Sound it with power and clarity. Take another breath and sound it again holding it for as long as you can. Note how the power of it increases. Feel yourself putting out beautiful, clear energy, wonderful loving sound, healing vibrations to all the universe. Sound your note with pride. Let the universe hear you. Make yourself truly heard. In this single sound put your truth and integrity out to the world.

This exercise can help you change your whole life if you work at it alongside the other new and healing practices you're developing.

Exercise 4

You'll need your notebook and about half an hour of uninterrupted time. Most of us don't have all the things we would like but that's often because we don't really know what we want. Now I'd like you to spend a few minutes looking at what would be perfect for you in terms of a home, career, relationship, etc. What do you really want? Try to crystallize your ideas and write them down. You'll probably need to add to them as time goes on and you become more comfortable about asking for what you want (see Cadillac vs. Volkswagen, p. 181).

From the prose you write, make affirmations that are positive statements in the present tense. If, for example, you've written, "I want a house in the country with a white picket fence and a paddock in the back for my horse," then the affirmation becomes, "I have a house in the country . . . etc."

I've been working on myself for many years, but I still do my affirmations every day. They cover every aspect of my life—my health, relationships, home, work, prosperity—everything. I have a stack of affirmation books that I've filled over the years and every now and then I have a look at them and see what I've created and give thanks for the way my life has developed. I always date them and I may work on a particular area for several days or even weeks until I achieve what I want (or something better), then I may move on to something else.

Some things always remain and are a kind of litany that I recite several times a day, often when I'm in a traffic jam or can't get on with whatever else I'm doing. I may say or write the same thing many times, sometimes changing a word here and there that will give it more meaning. I always end with a statement that Shakti Gawain uses in her book, *Creative Visualization*: "These things or something better are manifesting in my life now," and then I say some words of gratitude because I know that already these things are manifesting in my life though, for the present, they may be just beyond my view.

The Meditations

Meditation 1

Go to your safe place, take the phone off the hook and give yourself an hour or so to do this meditation. As usual, get comfortable, focus on your breathing and then let go of anything negative.

When you're relaxed, take your focus back to the age of fifteen or sixteen. You're going to collect together in a parcel the years from then until you were twenty-one. You don't need to see all the details unless you particularly

want to bring them to mind. In any case, know that whatever happened to you then is only a memory. You've already survived. Nothing from then can hurt you now. Take your time.

Now send love and light from your heart and wrap it around your self of that time. Hold and protect yourself tenderly, gently. Hold securely and with love just as you needed to be held then. And if you're able, send light and forgiveness to cleanse and heal that time.

Move to a higher spiritual level. Perhaps you can see that the people who did whatever they did then, including you, did so because of their own process and where they were in their lives at that time. They were living through their own damage and their own pain. And now, if you can, send them forgiveness with compassion. Free yourself and them once and for all. Let it go.

Now, if you are able, move into the third phase. Raise yourself to yet a higher spiritual level and look again. Maybe now you can see that those who were part of your life then were teaching you lessons you'd set for yourself to learn. They were helping you be more complete, as you were simultaneously helping them. Now, if you can, send forgiveness with love, compassion and gratitude to them and to yourself. Set them free. Let them go.

Now you are free of that time—let the past be healed.

When you're ready, give thanks to whatever higher power you believe in.

Allow your adolescent and young adult self to re-enter your heart and feel a sense of peace and wholeness. Stay for as long as you wish. When you're ready, gently begin to return to your physical being. Feel your toes and move them. Move your fingers. Gently stretch.

When you feel that you're back to the place behind your eyes, gently be aware of and thankful for your physical presence. Love your physical body. Open your eyes and return fully to the room.

Have a drink of water and record whatever you wish in your notebook.

Meditation 2

Go to your safe place, take the phone off the hook and get comfortable. Have your crystals, oils and perhaps a blue flower or two close by. Use the usual method to get relaxed and let go of anything negative.

Now, gently take your focus down to your throat, to the front of your neck, and with your eyes closed, visualize that area. See there a beautiful clear blue light. Cool but vibrant blue. Translucent, shining, clear blue.

See that light shining out. Out into the distance. Out in all directions. See it going out to all. Sending light to the world, to the higher selves of others. Shining, clear, healing light. Like a searchlight, clearing paths of communication. Down this wonderful path of light, send out loving messages to the world. Send out powerful loving, healing communication with the knowledge and conviction that every thought you think in this moment of clarity will be received by whoever is its target.

Send out mind messages, telepathically communicate with love and clarity. Send out messages to the universe beyond this planet, across the horizons of time and space to all the good there is now and all the good there is to come, to all the good there ever was. Send out a powerful message of love and gratitude and desire for communication and love. Clear your true path now.

CADILLAC VS. VOLKSWAGEN

Visualize exactly what you want and don't be afraid to ask for it.

I can't remember where I heard the following little tale, but I've used it often in workshops and most people find it both amusing and useful. I hope I'll be forgiven for not having permission to tell it.

A man died and went to heaven. He was met at the gate and was being escorted down the driveway, when his companion apologized for the fact that there were piles of brand new material goods along the pathway.

"I'm so sorry," he said, "but we ran out of space to store all these things that we have ready for people and then they just don't want them."

"I can't imagine anyone refusing these wonderful things," the man said. "Just look at that Cadillac over there. Why would anyone ever refuse that?"

"Well it's interesting that you should mention that," his escort replied, "because that was prepared for you."

"But I would never have refused that," the man said, astonished.

"But in your prayers, you kept asking for a Volkswagen," the escort replied. "So that's what we gave you."

It pays to know what you really want.

Now, allow any information that's for your higher good to enter into your throat chakra, down this beautiful path of blue light. Wisdom about your vocation, wisdom about your way forward, wisdom about your ultimate truth. Let the information simply flow in. Be the passive recipient of it without thinking or trying to make it happen or work it out in any way.

Now, switch on your tape recorder or pick up your notebook and pen. Open your throat and speak your message. Just let it flow without interruption, without self-consciousness. Let the wisdom that's flowing be captured forever.

When you feel you have caught on tape or on the page all you have to say for now, put down your recorder or pad.

Close your eyes again and, if necessary, get relaxed again. With a single thought, allow all your chakras to open. Draw the power of each to this point—the stability of your first, the flexibility of the second. The power and potential of the solar plexus and the love of the heart. The vision of the brow chakra and the understanding of the crown. Draw them all to this point and allow the combined power to come to your throat.

Now, open your throat. Allow the whole power of your being to issue forth on a single note. Let it come out on a breath. Hold it as long as you can then take another deep breath and again let your voice be heard. Let your vibration reach out to the farthest corners of the universe. Know that as the sound moves out into the world everything is changed by it. The vibration spreads out to touch everything and the love you send with it will touch the whole world. Repeat as often as you wish and when you're ready allow the sound to cease but know that the reverberation will go on forever.

Be silent in your space and allow the voice of the universe to speak to you. Hear that inner voice as it speaks to you in love.

Stay as long as you wish, and before you begin your return, give thanks.

When you're ready, begin your return to the room. With a thought, allow your chakras to close to where they are safe and comfortable.

Begin to be aware of your physical presence. Feel your fingers and toes. Move them a little. Gently stretch. Love your body and when you're back to that place behind your eyes, gently open your eyes and return to the room. Have a drink of water and record anything you wish in your notebook.

NINE

The Brow Chakra:
A Way Forward with Wisdom

～

Our deepest fear is not that we are inadequate. Our deepest fear is that we are powerful beyond measure. It is our light, not our darkness that most frightens us. We ask ourselves, who am I to be brilliant, gorgeous, talented and fabulous? Actually, who are you not to be?

You are a child of God. Your playing small doesn't benefit the world. There's nothing enlightened about shrinking so that other people won't feel insecure around you. We were born to make manifest the glory of God that is within us. It's not just in some of us, it's in everyone!

And as we let our light shine, we unconsciously give other people the permission to do the same. As we are liberated from our own fear, our presence automatically liberates others.

—Nelson Mandela, Inaugural speech, 1994

The higher we reach, the more quiet and gentle is the power and the more liberated we feel. The Sanskrit name for this chakra, *Anja*, means to command and it is here that we finally take command of our life.

The brow chakra orchestrates all we have thus far perceived and molds it into a pleasing symphony. Although our whole ascent has been helping us take our life into our own hands and drive it forward, here we can really make that possible in a magical way. This is the place of manifestation and miracles.

The awakening of this chakra, with its gifts of inspiration, insight, perception, wisdom and vision, can lift us to unimaginable ecstasy. It offers gifts we may only have dreamed of, or indeed of gifts we may never have dared dream of. But they are the gifts that children's dreams are made of. Magical things. The things we could conceive of when we were young, while we still remembered what powerful spirits we are, when all things were possible. Before we were told to put away such flights of fancy and get our feet on the ground. Before education, science and rational thought took over.

Here you can revisit some of those dreams and, with your feet firmly planted in the stabilizing energy of the earth, your root chakra taking care of your need to remain in your physical being, you can explore again the joys of expanded vision and thought. Allow yourself to soar into the realms of the spirit. Here you can see beyond physical seeing, hear beyond human hearing, use intuition beyond rational explanation.

You can add to your daily life by living simultaneously on two planes. The overall outcome is that your spiritual life becomes such second nature that all transactions are more stimulating and joyous, all experience more rich and vibrant and life takes on a new wonder as you become aware of the learning available in every single event in life. It becomes a challenge to look at why you are going down a different road because you missed your usual turning while driving to work; why someone who was crossing the road when you were stopped at the red light looked deep into your eyes and you'll never forget that look; why someone appears hostile and jealous; or why life has brought you to this place.

Throughout this journey our accent has been on forgiving the past so we don't go on carrying old and unnecessary baggage. Now we can see at a glance that the only way forward was to be where we were, and we can forgive and understand. For now we're blessed with the wisdom of all our experiences so far. Although the greatest understanding is yet to come at the seventh chakra, here is wisdom beyond anything that can be taught, beyond intellectual knowledge, beyond academic learning. Do you know some people who, despite the fact that they may have left school early, or had little opportunity for academic training, are nevertheless the people you would like to sit and listen to for hours? They appear to speak from a different perspective, and wisdom just rolls off their tongues, often in a colorful and picturesque way as they use analogy and example drawn from a wide experience of life?

My father was one of these. I could listen to him for hours as he drew amazing insights from the most simple of stories. I have met people like that all over the world. Old women in Africa, who in the simplest of language would reveal wisdom that could change your life. Such wisdom demonstrates an open and unobstructed sixth chakra. Laurens van der Post in his wonderful books *A Story like the Wind* and *A Far Off Place* used this kind of wisdom, also in an African setting, as a means of transmitting the wonderful messages those books carry.

If you look again at the diagram of the caduceus (see page 68), you'll see that there's a central staff around which two snakes coil. In symbolic terms this staff represents the central energy channel, the *sushumna*, and the two snakes the two more lateral channels, the *ida* and *pingala* (see Glossary). The uppermost point where all three meet is the representation of the sixth chakra. This is the first of two chakras located in the head, both in direct contact with the brain and closely linked.

Sometimes erroneously called the third eye, the brow chakra is located above and between the physiological eyes. It is the chakra of seeing, not only in practical, physiological terms, but in the deeper sense of inner vision and intuition. It's the place of insight—in-sight, inner vision. The brow chakra brings all the others together in readiness for the final ascent to the crown where our spirituality may finally reach full bloom.

Magic, Miracles and Manifestation

Here once again we can return to the magic of childhood, to unlimited possibilities, to skills we have always had but which were drowned by life. Now we rediscover them and refine them. We are reintroduced to our true power as spiritual beings.

Although the revelations of the lower chakras, if you have continued to work on them, will have changed your life, it's here that the magic becomes reality. It's in the clearing and development of this chakra that we move to the point where we learn to manifest material things almost with a thought. It's with a thought that we can send out powerful healing, that we can change our own lives and be a model to help those around us. Be inspired, for here you can begin to have whatever your mind and heart desires.

We learned about the power of affirmation in the previous chapter, and how we can truly change our lives by repeating them, readjusting them until they fit and feel right. Of course, we must still do the other chakra work also but the brow takes manifestation a stage further. I'm not suggesting that you stop doing the work (and, as I said, I still do my affirmations every day), but as the brow opens, things suddenly become easier. Life flows in an even more amazing way. The secret is in being open to the flow of spirit. When we are in this state, anything can happen as we project powerful images into the world and make them our reality.

Shakti Gawain moved a whole generation to a new understanding of personal empowerment with her beautiful little book, *Creative Visualization*. Since then visualization has become widely used in the everyday life of many. It is now recognized as a powerful therapeutic tool in the treatment of illness. For example, visualization of healthy cells overtaking and destroying cancer cells can help arrest the illness; visualizing bronchioles opening when feeling wheezy can help asthmatics avert an attack. All of us can improve every area of our life by visualization.

Many athletes use the technique of visualizing themselves playing their shot perfectly and some will refuse to proceed until they've rehearsed in their mind several times how they want the game to go. A controlled study of basketball players proved beyond doubt that those who visualized themselves winning the game could improve their performance even without actual practice. Just think what a difference you could make to your life by spending a little time on this (see the end of the chapter for exercises).

Seeing, Clairvoyance and Vision

This is the chakra of seeing. It's here that we begin to awaken and clarify our inner vision. Stimulated by the opening of our creativity at the sacral chakra, enhanced at the throat, now we add vision to have a clear picture of what we want our lives to be. Pulling together vision, creative thought, good heart, pure intention and confidence, we can make our lives happen.

The universe, by synchronicity of events, nudges us forward to where we are meant to be and if we are wise, we follow. Although we always have free choice, we need to bear in mind that we are here for a reason and generally we cannot with impunity stray far from the path we are supposed to tread.

If I am meant to work in one place doing a particular thing, that's where I'll be. The universe will somehow lead me there, and if I'm sensible I'll follow the signposts. When at times I've tried to ignore those signposts and do it my way, I've had a kick from the universe to get me back on track. I can make my journey much more enjoyable, rewarding and fun by working with the universe. I can produce what I want as long as what I ask for is for my higher good and the higher good of all. This is where my inner vision comes in. And the visions I have need not only be for me. I can have visions for the world: for example, of everyone being so empowered by love that we don't need to worry about closing down our chakras anymore; of a solution to poverty; of universal esteem and respect so that armed conflict can be replaced by negotiation and peace.

I can have a multitude of visions, some of them tiny and to be fulfilled in an instant and others that may need to be part of a group vision if they are to become reality. But whatever they are, they can begin to change things quite powerfully from the moment they are conceived. To be a visionary is a great gift to the world. Why not close your eyes and create a great vision for the planet right now?

The brow chakra also allows us a different kind of seeing. Usually we can only see the external contours of physical manifestations. For example, I can see a closed box and perceive its shape, its color and texture, but I can't generally see inside it unless its walls are transparent. You can see the shape and form of your friends, but generally not what is going on inside them in a physical sense. We are limited to this view because that is all we think we're capable of seeing. But why shouldn't you be able to see more? All that stops you from doing so is a collection of molecules that are placed in such a way as to apparently block the view. If you've trained your mind to manifest what you've told it to, why then can't you train it to pass through this veil of molecules?

Development of the sixth chakra allows you to see beyond, and with some practice you can learn to look inside. There are healers who are particularly gifted in this way. They can diagnose by inner vision and then channel healing using the brow chakra and, of course, an open crown and heart. Barbara Brennan gives a beautiful account of inner vision in her book *Hands of Light*.

Though the natural development of this chakra occurs between the ages of twenty-one and twenty-six, some never develop it in this lifetime. Also, it may be that you'll need to revisit this chakra many times before you perfect such a gift. Many of the spiritual gifts I mentioned in the last chapter and here do not develop until we revisit our chakras in our forties and fifties.

Perhaps the most well-known gift following the stimulation of the sixth chakra is that of clairvoyance, clear sight, which allows us to see beyond the horizons of time and space. This is a gift with practical implications, whether to help us locate lost articles or people, to glimpse a different time or simply to help us see everything more clearly. As with all these gifts, anyone can learn to use clairvoyance to some degree given time and the will to work on it.

The Time Continuum

At this level, we're confronted with the concept of time and what that means. The seasons, night and day and the cycle of the moon remind us of the cyclical nature of all things natural. So is time simply a man-made system to help us organize our lives and have consistent communication? To enable us to understand each other when we talk in terms of hours, days, weeks and years?

Really time exists as a continuum. So why shouldn't it be possible to view it all at once? If we took off the blinkers of education, tradition and self-imposed limitations, could we, from the vantage point of this single moment, look in both directions along that continuum and see with clarity both the past and the future? Or indeed may we find that the whole of time is in this moment?

The brow chakra simply enables us to flatten out the mountains that usually prevent us from seeing beyond the horizons of time and space and to use this information for our highest good.

You may already have started to become more aware of the past, even the very distant past, as we've come along our journey. You may have found yourself having an occasional breakthrough of past experience, either from this lifetime or even from an earlier one. For instance, you may have started to feel particularly attracted to a certain place or time in history. Or you may have met people who you feel you've known before, or maybe forever—and probably you have. Such karmic connections are not uncommon.

Because we're conditioned to think quite naturally in terms of memories and remembering things, such experiences are much easier to accept than glimpses of the future, even though these past life snapshots are much more than mere memory. The past, as I've said before, is for us to learn from, nothing more. If you have found yourself having a lot of such experiences, it might be an idea for you to gently address them, maybe by doing a past-life workshop. These often show us reasons for current behavior patterns and present relationships, especially if the patterns happen to be destructive and repetitive.

It can be beneficial to go back and heal the past so that we can at last let go of something we've carried into this lifetime. But if you decide to do so, make sure you choose a very skilled guide who can hold both you and the situation and heal anything that comes up.

Some would say there is enough for us to deal with in this lifetime without looking elsewhere. And for many that's true. However, for some, the answers to this life's difficulties are easy to unveil and heal by searching through the past. So if, while reading this, you have a genuine curiosity tempered with a light excited feeling about having such an experience, perhaps you would benefit from a past life regression.

And the future? That is also simply a continuation of time, and if we look in the right way it isn't so difficult to view. Please remember what I said earlier about not using such gifts as party games. Any excursion in time should be for ourselves and for the higher good of all. Unless you're working professionally as a clairvoyant, it would be wise for you to confine yourself to planning and manifesting your own future.

Different Types of Memory

Memory is governed by the brow chakra and it may be that as you clear this area, there's a flood of long-forgotten memories. If, as you practice the exercises, these are painful, remember that you have survived the reality and will now survive the memory. However, treat yourself with gentleness and compassion and share the experience with that trusted person we talked about in Chapter 2 (A Sympathetic Ear).

Memory is so much part of our everyday life that we hardly think about it unless, for some reason, we start to have difficulties in remembering. Memory operates in three stages: initially we must concentrate enough to lay down a memory trace in the first place (quite often what appears to be a problem of memory is really a problem of concentration); at the second stage we organize and store the memory; and the third stage is that of recalling information when we need it.

Then there's short-term and long-term memory. We remember facts that we learned as children. That's long term. And also what we had for breakfast, or a phone number someone just gave us. That's short term. Often as people get older they begin to lose short-term memory while still being able to recount wonderful stories of their childhood.

These are intellectual memories. However, there are also physical memories. For example, my body has stored memory in its tissues. It may react to a particular situation even though I don't remember it intellectually. An example of this is the pelvic numbness often felt by women who've suffered sexual abuse, whenever they try to make love. Then there are feeling memories, such as when I feel anxious or afraid in a certain situation even though I have no intellectual memory of ever having been there before. The intellectual memory has been repressed, but the feelings remain. Being aware of these different types and levels of memory can help us sort out what's happened to us in the past and what we need to heal.

Using Your Intuition

We discovered that we become aware of our gut feelings at the solar plexus. These feelings are now refined to intuition at the brow chakra.

Intuition is a handy sixth sense which is often half mocked as a female attribute, i.e. "feminine intuition." This is probably because in the past it was exhibited more commonly by women, who are less likely than men to feel self-conscious about acting on something that defies scientific proof.

Intuition is, in fact, a function of the right side of the brain, the so-called feminine side wherein lies the feminine principle. But, as I said in Chapter 5, the evolved being has such a good balance of the masculine and the feminine that such a gift can be exhibited just as expertly by men.

Rational thought and logic are governed by the left (masculine) side of the brain. Sadly, a modern education that encourages the search for proof often leads to the subduing of the more creative, feminine gifts, intuition being one of them. I certainly have suffered ridicule throughout my career when, despite facts pointing to the contrary, I've gone with my gut feelings and treated someone the way my intuition, reinforced by other spiritual gifts, has dictated. That's not to say I haven't gone on to carry out modern investigation to confirm my intuitive diagnosis. The point is that we can offer the best to ourselves and everyone else if we integrate the scientific and the spiritual.

I've often said that if someone called me and asked me to meet them at King's Cross station at one o'clock and my intuition said Waterloo station at two, then I'd go to Waterloo. It's not quite as clear cut as that, however. There are many factors at play, not least of which is our mood. If I'm in a space where I'm finely tuned and working, then I follow my intuition implicitly.

I can use intuition accurately for diagnosis and to embark on a course of treatment long before scientific proof is available to back my hunch. I can tune in at the beginning of someone's history and trace exactly what has happened to them before they tell me the rest. However, I can also totally overrule my intuition when I want to do something, and I can miss the most obvious facts about people when I want to believe the best about them—the latter more often in my personal rather than my professional life. The moral is that our intuition is a very useful tool that can be honed to perfection, but sometimes we forget or neglect to use it.

Healing

Healing is what this book's all about, and there are many levels at which it can occur. It can be as simple as helping yourself or someone else find some peace within themselves and as dramatic as arresting hemorrhage or mending fractured limbs.

Healing in the formal sense, as practiced by healers, needs open heart and crown chakras as well as the vision that comes from the brow. The higher you go up the chakra system, the more your own healing powers will awaken.

A word of caution. Channeling healing for someone without their permission is an assault! Only in cases of dire emergency, for example at the scene of an accident, may we dispense with the need to have the patient's permission. Just because we may feel we're doing something loving and beautiful doesn't mean it's acceptable to everyone. Each of us has a right to decide how we wish to be treated and, except in very special circumstances, no one has a right to overrule someone's wishes.

Of course, the person receiving healing can also block the energy to a great extent, but that isn't the point. If you feel you have a vocation to be a healer, please go and have some proper training at a reputable school. Such training will always include work on ethics.

It's been said that with pure heart and good intention you can't do any harm, but that's not altogether true. I remember an alternative practitioner who, while being retained to do one piece of work with one of my patients, began to do some hands-on healing without the patient's consent and without warning. The result was quite disastrous. Events we'd been working on very slowly and carefully came hurtling to the fore and the novice practitioner was totally incapable of dealing with them. Though some would say that what was there needed to come up and be dealt with, what was also needed was someone expert enough to handle the emergence of the pain. The moral is: please don't mess with anything unless you're invited, properly trained and supervised. It's quite a different matter holding your child and flowing love into him/her in order to help, or indeed projecting love into a situation that obviously needs it. But if in doubt, don't meddle!

Sending Mind Messages

This section might be termed elementary telepathy. However, such a name seems to shroud in a kind of mystique something that we do spontaneously many times a day.

Telepathy is the picking up of information from one mind to the other without the stimulus of speech or hearing. It is a gift we receive at the throat chakra but which is honed at the brow. We can learn to do this more formally if someone is willing to be a transmitter and another the receiver.

There are times when we have all wanted to talk to someone and while thinking about them, they call. There are other times when people who know each other well can pick up distressing mind messages from each other. On a journey in the United States I was talking to a young man who told me he'd been ill some time previously and was in a place in Africa where communication wasn't particularly easy. His mother had been in Scandinavia at a conference and suddenly she knew she had to leave and fly home even though no one had been able to contact her. The more clear our brow chakra, the easier such communication is. Like all spiritual gifts it's open to abuse and shouldn't be used without the permission of the other, except in cases such as those I've mentioned. The best rule of thumb is to ask yourself how you'd like it if someone did the same to you. I dare say you'd feel violated, and so would I. Though, most of the time I'm happy to share my thoughts, they're the most private thing I have and I have a right to keep it that way.

Inspiration

Sometimes when working with people on their affirmations or getting them to find out what they really want, I tune in to them, asking them to change a word here and there to subtly change the meaning until I can see and feel them come into alignment. Something clicks and suddenly all their chakras are open at once, balanced and aligned. Something changes in the eyes—they have become inspired, in-spirit. They've formed a connection to a higher energy and now that they've experienced that feeling, they'll never forget it. It's difficult to describe, but once you've felt it you'll know what you are aiming for in future.

For me it comes with a feeling of excitement and a rush of energy. Suddenly everything is crystal clear and I know it's right. Gently it almost lifts me off my feet and I hardly dare breathe for a moment.

Then I relax into it and there it is, a running stream of energy as the spirit pours through me and all possible doubt about the wisdom of what I'm doing or saying is gone. It's similar to my feeling of spirituality that I described in Chapter 3.

Having reached this point, we become aware of an internal shift that gives us a totally new and inspiring connection with the divine, whatever that may be for each of us. There is a new reverence, almost a tearful joy coupled with excitement as we approach this point. It's at the brow that we begin to feel devotion.

Sometimes in focusing on the divine, we can hardly breathe—and we don't seem to need to. It's the most wonderful feeling of never-ending love washing over and through and swirling all around. It gives me a strange, exciting but slightly uncomfortable feeling in my tummy as I'm almost overwhelmed by the power and absolute joy of it. This is devotion.

It's different from my deep and intense love for my partner, my children, my parents. It's qualitatively different and almost shocking in its intensity. This is my love for God. I can't describe it more fully. I can only hope that you can feel it for yourself, because when you do, you'll know that whatever you need in this life, whatever difficulties you may have, all can be resolved. No obstacle can stand in your way now. You have cleared the path and you have direct access to God.

You may become aware of great souls around you. Of amazing presences who are there to welcome you and help you to carry the love to all those you meet. You may be flooded with ideas, with energy, with wisdom, with knowledge, or you may be transfixed and simply held in love and peace. There are many ways in which this wonderful state manifests for me, but no matter how differently it may present, it's undeniably the same thing. I'm flooded with gratitude for all things.

From this place I can send unlimited love and healing. Not only to all those who are sick and in need but to the whole universe. I can send out a powerful message of love, asking that it will fall where it's needed most. From this point with all my chakras open and clear, I can radiate love with all my heart, my soul, my might. I can send powerful unconditional loving to wherever it is needed. I can send healing, gentle but powerful healing to all the planet. I can send messages of spiritual love out from the planet to the universe beyond so that all other life forms may feel the love there is here. I can send love back in time to heal the past and forward to heal the future. I can send love along the continuum of time, bursting out like a million stars into the ether. I can send love and healing in shooting beams of light. In streams and raging rivers. I send it with power and with gentleness, in tiny trickles of light and in lasers so powerful they can cut through any darkness. I send love that can heal the world. I send this devotion that opens up all possibilities and renders my life, my spirit, my love endless. And I thank God.

All we have been doing thus far is a kind of prayer. It's practical loving, forgiving, striving to make life better for ourselves and others. That's prayer.

As we've seen, those who have spiritual or religious beliefs are much more likely to do well after illness or surgery. Prayer in a formal sense, either alone or with a congregation of others, can be not only comforting, but can have real benefits for the quality of life of those who participate.

Prayer in a much less formal sense also adds a completely different dimension to life. What do you think would happen if instead of praying in words you visualized all that you were praying for? Not only what you want to have, but also in gratitude for all that you already have. If instead of making a list, you could actually see yourself in the perfect life, the perfect situation—feel it, touch it, smell it, be it. See yourself glowing with good health and energy, with love in your life, your body strong with lots of stamina, with friends who are there for you but give you space, in a calm and peaceful home, doing what you love to do and being secure financially. Imagine it, visualize it, feel it and give thanks for it. It's all entering your life right now even though you can't quite see it yet. It's just beyond those horizons of time and space.

Working with Color

We can't leave this chakra of vision without mentioning color. This is something I used to neglect, but it only took a single session with a dear friend and colleague (Theo Gimbel of the Hygeia College of Color Therapy near Stroud, England) to convince me not only of its efficacy as a therapy, but also of its great diagnostic possibilities in the hands of an expert.

A very simple but effective self-diagnostic test is the Luscher Color Test. It certainly can't take the place of a professional assessment or therapy, but its accuracy about your personality and where you are now in life may amaze you. Hopefully it will whet your appetite for more.

Our journey through the chakras has touched on the colors associated with each energy center, and a great deal can be done to help clear them by just wearing something of the color of the chakra you're working on. If you're having difficulty with communication for example, a beautiful blue scarf could well help. If you can't find much joy in your life and are held back with old bitterness or anger, try something yellow. Red will help you realize your power and help you assert your will, whereas green or pink will aid you in being gentle and loving. Purple is a good color for healers to wear (one of my favorites), as is bright but deep blue, which opens up my brow chakra and aids intuition, healing and clairvoyance. If you're having difficulty with your sexuality or relationships, have something orange around you. You'll find that changing your color scheme at home can profoundly affect everything from your mood to your relationships and your prosperity.

Dysfunction at the Brow Chakra

This chakra can function quite well in some of its aspects even if it is underdeveloped and blocked. You can have a rational, bright, lively and highly analytical mind but without the embellishments of wisdom, self-awareness and the ability to transcend rational thought. Traditional education often dulls intuition and creativity, and without the sensitivity of the brow chakra may lead to an intellectual arrogance that undervalues all but what can be scientifically proven.

I know a man who is intellectually stimulating, his academic brilliance second to none. His memory is sharp, his wit sardonic and potentially cruel. As long as he isn't crossed, he can appear to be supportive, friendly and kind. However, he's driven by his competitive nature, his greed for money and his lack of inner security. His intellectual arrogance renders him incapable of the sensitivity required to see the other person's point of view, to allow freedom and to respect beliefs that are not in line with his own. He is so threatened by the fact that he may not remain in control. Though for a while he appears to have people's respect, ultimately he's surrounded either by sycophants or by those who are afraid of him.

This man typifies the blocking of the sixth chakra, although of course this isn't his only difficulty. But because he performs well in many areas and is unaware of the damage he creates around him, he's unlikely ever to agree to do the spiritual work that could completely transform his life. He's one of those I mentioned in discussing prosperity who may appear to be prosperous but who are not in the true sense of the word. All they have is a lot of money.

Blocks here generally render the person unable to follow through with the creative ideas they have. Such people appear to be surrounded by plans that never quite come to completion. They either seem to be unaware of this, almost forgetting what they suggested they'd do and being unaware of the frustration they cause others, or else they project the frustration they feel as their lives become clogged with half-fulfilled plans. They then tend to blame others for their own shortcomings. Although they may be very bright, they never quite reach their potential in the broadest sense since their vision is either stunted or negative, and they only perform well in an environment where they can assume a great degree of control. They're never quite able to feel the kind of joy we mentioned earlier and are inclined to ridicule those who can. They can be quite cruel in their desire to put others down, to trample on finer emotions and to prove that their negative view of the world is correct. Sometimes if their world becomes threatened either by illness of a loved one or by loss, they unblock very quickly and may then become quite zealous in their new-found "religion," though even then they may have difficulty surrendering to the work they really need to do to change their lives completely. There is usually an accompanying crown chakra problem and they really don't know what we're talking about when we speak in spiritual terms.

Do protect yourself if you know someone like this. They're often very powerful, very bright and quite affable, and at first may seduce you as they articulate their ideas. But they're likely to deny what you thought had been agreed, fail to honor commitments and leave you questioning your own sanity.

In the physical sense, the area most affected by a sixth chakra block is vision, and there may be eye strain, conjunctivitis, poor sight or blindness. Headaches and migraine may occur and there may be difficulties with memory. In this chakra more than any other, there may be little if any physical manifestation of the problem, though sometimes nightmares may give a clue.

UNANSWERED PRAYERS

There's a song by Garth Brooks with the refrain, "and I thank God for unanswered prayers." I'm sure we all have some of them. When I first returned to England from Africa I didn't quite know what to do with myself because I was in a state of shock, having lost my home, my way of life and much that was dear to me. I interviewed for a job that was well paid, part-time and very close to home. I really wanted it because it seemed to fulfill all my needs right then. I failed at the second interview and was very disappointed. However, within a few months I'd changed my life beyond all recognition and had embarked on a new career in psychiatry away from surgery, which had been my first love. I often think back to then and give thanks for not having gotten what I so desperately begged for. It certainly wouldn't have been for my higher good!

The Exercises

The oils that are particularly useful for work at this chakra are violet and rose geranium. Why not burn one of these in your vaporizer as you proceed with the work?

There are four stones that are wonderful for opening and clarifying the brow. My favorite, which I wear every day, is amethyst. Not only does it cleanse, strengthen, energize and protect, it brings about spiritual enhancement, cuts through illusion, and strengthens inspiration, divine love and intuition. Just imagine all that. How could you bear to be without it?

The second, celestite—a beautiful stone—is useful for both brow and throat since it aids inspiration, accelerates spiritual growth and makes us more aware of divine intervention while also helping us with creative expression.

Alexandrite isn't easy to find and even a tiny piece can be quite expensive. However, it's powerful yet gentle, helping us balance mind, body and spirit and feel joy and love again if we're recovering from any kind of serious trauma. Here at the brow it helps open and clarify our inner vision as does the last stone of my choice, the Herkimer diamond, a clear, bright crystal that isn't as expensive as it sounds.

With whatever oil or stone you wish to use, or indeed with a deep blue flower or a piece of deep blue or purple cloth, go to your safe place with your notebook, giving yourself plenty of uninterrupted time. Begin as you always do with your breathing, relaxing your body and letting go of anything negative.

Exercise 1

Close your eyes and imagine a clear crystal screen. It is free from any other image. If any object appears on it before you're ready, just gently allow it to slide away again.

On that screen, I'd like you to create your ideal world. This is like a movie screen, so the picture can change whenever you want it to, but

I'd like you to start with any area of your life—perhaps your home, your career, your special relationship—and visualize it in every detail. You can see the whole picture just as you want it to be. Allow it to develop before your eyes and change it if you want to until you feel it's just right. Can you see the colors, the tiniest of details, hear the birds singing if there are any in your vision, or the music playing? Is the sun shining? Are there clouds in the sky? Does your ideal home have a garden? Is there a pet playing there? Are you wealthy? Is it a large home or somewhere small and cozy? Is it light and airy or does it have soft lights and a mysterious air?

And your ideal job—where is it? What are you doing? Is it in an office or working outside? Is it with other people or in a studio alone? What are you wearing? What are you feeling? Watch the scene as you make it perfect for you.

Your perfect relationship? Are you married or living with someone or enjoying your solitude while having someone special to be with when you choose to do so? Is it a sexual relationship or one that's close and mutually supportive without the need for sexual intimacy? Is it with someone of the opposite sex or is it a same-sex relationship? What's right for you? See it and feel it and remember it.

In this moment send a prayer in whatever form you wish with absolute confidence that, as long as you're asking for something that will truly benefit you and not harm anyone else, you can have that or something better.

Give thanks.

Stay with your crystal screen for as long as you wish, and when you're ready to return, make a note that you'll remember all of this in all its detail or go back and find more when you wish. And now, ground yourself, then return to the room, take your notebook and describe your perfect world.

As you do so, affirm it. You may find yourself automatically making affirmations as you go since that process is becoming second nature to you now. When you've finished, send out thanks to wherever you want to send them.

Know that you can return to your vision to make it real, make it happen, continue to affirm it and create what you really want in your life. Don't be surprised if your vision has changed from when you began to work on yourself, or indeed if it continues to change now. What you might have thought you wanted some time ago may not seem so important now. You may have thought your perfect partner had a handsome face and brown eyes, only to find now that the most important features are loyalty, trustworthiness and a sense of humor and that the rest hardly matters anymore. Or that your need for lots of money in the bank has been replaced by good earning capacity and you see yourself supporting some worthwhile cause with the money you don't need.

You may also find that you already have much of your ideal world. It's been developing as you've continued on your journey and as you've done your daily affirmations. You have been doing your affirmations, haven't you? This would be a good time to go back and look at them and check off what you've already created. As always, give thanks.

Exercise 2

If you want to try out your clairvoyant skills, here's a way to start. This is just a little gentle fun, but if you want to develop this gift, I'd recommend that you have an assessment for a psychic unfoldment class and train properly.

Perhaps there's an object you can't find. That's where we'll begin. Have beside you a clear quartz crystal if you have one, but if not, it doesn't matter. The reason people use crystal balls is that it helps focus and clear your mind, but you've learned how to do that by now anyway.

Close your eyes and clear your mind—use the same crystal screen as in the last exercise if you like. Now, bring to mind the lost object. See it in as much detail as you can and place it on the crystal screen. Continue to focus on it and let a scene develop around it. See if you recognize what is developing. Watch it carefully. Take your time and try to let it develop without thinking about it or making it happen. Be very observant. You may find that you will suddenly recognize some of the scene—another object, a place. Can you see where it is? Don't lose heart if you can't do it the first time. Play with it a little and you'll find that the more you tell yourself you can do it, the easier it will become.

As always, give thanks and ground yourself before you return to the room.

Exercise 3

Now it's time for you to have some fun and spoil yourself a little. Why not look in the phone book, find a color consultant and make an appointment to go and have your colors read? You'll find this an exciting adventure that will change your energy, lift your mood, complement your natural coloring and improve your complexion so that you look much younger. Men as well as women, please.

It doesn't have to cost you a fortune and don't think that you suddenly have to throw out everything in your wardrobe that isn't the right color. You just tell your friends and family so that they can help you change direction a little, color-wise. When you buy new, you'll start to gradually replace things with what suits you better. But right now you deserve a treat, so you could buy yourself at least a little something new. A silk handkerchief? A new scarf? Enjoy yourself.

The Meditations

Meditation 1

Here we are at the point of vision, wisdom and command. We've come a long way on our journey and you're much clearer and healthier than you were when you began. There's always more work to do, however, until it's time for us to go home. So . . .

Take yourself off to your safe place with your flowers, your oils, your crystals or whatever you wish to take. Make yourself comfortable with as much support as you need to allow you to physically hold your position for a while.

Focus on your breathing and relax your body, letting go of anything negative through your base chakra and the soles of your feet. Feel yourself fill with love almost automatically as you adopt this pose. It's healing now just to be here. Enjoy that feeling. Know what you've accomplished to be able to connect so easily and feel the energy flow. Feel the peace. Feel the joy. Feel the love. Feel your spirituality.

Now, loving yourself, take yourself back to the age of twenty-one and allow yourself to send love and forgiveness to yourself and others and the events of that time. Let your mind wander with you until the age of about twenty-six and let the love you're flowing cleanse, heal and forgive that whole period.

Now, as you've done so many times before, raise yourself spiritually so you can see that whoever may have hurt you then was living out his or her own process, and forgive. Send love.

When you're ready, rise again to that highest level where not only can you forgive, but you can be grateful for the teaching that those experiences gave you. Take your time. Give thanks.

When you're ready, ground yourself. Start to be aware of your physical body. Move your toes and your fingers. Stretch and gently return to the room. Have a drink of water and record whatever you wish in your notebook. Take as much time as you wish before going on to the next meditation.

Meditation 2

Settle down into your safe place and induce that relaxed state in the usual way. Let go of anything negative through the soles of your feet and your root chakra.

Now, bring your focus to that place slightly above and between your eyebrows, to the point of your brow chakra. Feel that very spot and see it glowing with a wonderful deep bright blue light. With a single loving thought simply allow that whole area to be cleansed with light. See the light shine even more brightly now, deep, rich, dark blue, maybe with a purple tinge.

From behind that point of light at your forehead, and right through the center of it, shine a bright white light now. Shining out clear and strong, this light reaches beyond the horizons of time and space.

Whoever and whatever is in your life now came from far away. There were times when you couldn't see those who are close to you now. They were in a different time and a different place. They were walking into your life but you couldn't yet see them. They were making their way, as you were too, until you both came to a particular point in time and space where there was so little distance between you that you met. Now there are others who are also making their way toward you.

In this moment, clear your vision and look out down the wonderful light that is shining now through your brow. That light is a spotlight that shines out beyond the horizons of time and space. It shines to a place and time that you have not as yet been able to see, but that time and that space are peopled with those who are making their way into your life now just as surely as you are making your way toward them. They are people to bring you love and joy, hope and beauty, work and opportunity. They are the people of your future as you are one of the people of their future also.

Now, allow them to move toward you. Allow them to come into view. You may not be able to see their faces, but you can see their form. Watch them bringing wonderful gifts into your life as you are taking gifts to them.

Send out a beam of love to embrace them. Send out joy and hope. Send out a welcome and know that as the time and space between you diminish so you will welcome them and they will welcome you also.

These may be souls you have known forever. They may be souls you have never met but the fact that they are coming into your life means they are bringing you gifts in the form of love and growth and experience, which you need in order to continue on your own journey of spiritual growth. You have mutual lessons to give and receive. You can do it all with love.

Stay a while. Feel the wonderful energy between you. Enjoy the feeling of the love flowing out of you and of holding them in love.

But for the moment this is where you are, and they still belong a little distance from you. So now, send a final beam of love and a promise that when the time comes you will meet them in love, you will meet them with joy, you will meet them with openness, you will meet them with a sense of brotherhood and sisterhood, you will meet them as equals.

And now allow them to go. Let them recede to where they need to be in their lives right now.

Give thanks and gently allow the beam of love to be once more reabsorbed and begin on your return to the room. Be aware of your brow chakra and allow it to close to where it is most comfortable. You can open it again whenever you wish.

Be aware of your physical presence. Ground yourself. Gently move your fingers and your toes, and when you're ready, open your eyes. Take your time. Have a drink of water. Record whatever you wish in your notebook. Don't forget to put the phone back on the hook when you're ready.

TEN

The Crown Chakra: Crowning Our Spirituality

~

Behold, the mellow light that floods the eastern sky.
In signs of praise both heaven and earth unite.
And from the fourfold manifested powers a chant of love arises,
both from the flaming fire and the flowing water,
and from sweet smelling earth and from rustling wind,
from the deep unfathomable vortex of that golden light in which
the victor bathes,
all nature's worldless voice in a thousand tones arises to proclaim;
Joy unto you, O men of Earth.
A pilgrim has returned back from the other shore.
A conscious being is born.

—*Vedic tradition*

While writing *The Seven Healing Chakras*, I've sometimes thought ahead to how I would tackle this chapter on the crown chakra, since its wonder can't really be described in words. I could spend hours writing the longest chapter of the book, and still the only way for you to really feel what I'm trying to say is to experience it.

It's so limitless, so boundless, so lacking in any material substance and yet it encompasses everything in an instant. In a single glance from here I could be in Atlantis in one instant and the 21st century in the next. I can be there, feel, hear, visualize without any material change having taken place at all. I can create, perceive and experience from within in infinite detail, at infinite speed. I'm in a never-ending circle where there is only consciousness. Consciousness that makes everything possible. Consciousness that enables me to manifest all that I have. Consciousness that is invisible and yet visible in everything there is.

Kahlil Gibran uses a wonderful metaphor. He states, "Work is love made visible." Perhaps we could extend that. Manifestation is consciousness made visible. Here we are at the pinnacle of our journey, the moment we've been working for as at last we open to our crown. This is the chakra that was so carefully protected by the elaborate headdress of the ancient kings, and now by more modern monarchs with their crowns. This wearing of crowns comes from ancient times when kings were seen as gods.

The god-kings of ancient Egypt's statues still inspire awe today as they stand hundreds of feet tall, their apparel protecting all their chakras carved in stone. In the ancient art and craft of most cultures and in religious art over the centuries there is acknowledgment of the chakras, but even where reference to all the other chakras has been lost the crown chakra remains, usually depicted as a halo.

Here we come to understanding, universal truth and knowledge and from here we can learn to transcend all we have known thus far. From here we can program ourselves to reach the unreachable, to touch the untouchable and to find, initially only for tiny snatches of time, absolute peace where everything is suspended and we have utter awareness. We are in ecstasy.

When we learn to hold this state for longer and eventually to live it simultaneously with our human life, we are permanently changed and for the most part can be calm and serene. Something wondrous happens to us. We have glimpsed heaven, have experienced bliss; we're transformed and we can never be the same again. And when we're working with the energy of the crown, we radiate love and peace to all those around us. Though this takes time, dedication and patience, it is worth every bit of effort. But don't forget that even when we've reached that place we remain ordinary human beings, doing ordinary things with our feet on the ground.

This final step can free us totally from depression and apathy, fear and confusion, and bring us to awareness and a clear state of consciousness.

Knowledge and Truth

We talked of truth at our throat chakra and here we meet it again. Universal truth exists as a single solitary state. All the truth there ever was and will be exists in a single moment.

We touched on the fact that we're all on the path to universal truth and are simply at different points on that path, approaching it from different angles, collecting like pilgrims at the Mecca of truth and knowledge. That is our primary goal: to come to a point of knowing, of enlightenment, of being at one again with the great body of God.

Just as the truth exists, so does knowledge. All the knowledge there ever was and ever will be already exists. As a seed contains the whole template of the plant and the strand of DNA holds the key to the whole person, this moment holds all the truth. We have only to find it. We are usually taking small bites of truth as we focus on one particular aspect of knowledge. We digest it and then bite off another piece. And as we grow we refine and retune what we know, discarding the elementary form we knew previously in favor of the finer detail.

But here at the crown, we're suddenly able to be free of the constraints of our human brain and can immerse ourselves in the truth as we transcend and have a connection with the divine source. Here at last we can understand as we surrender to that which is so much greater than us and yet of which we are a powerful part.

At this point in our development we're called upon to re-dedicate our lives to whatever we feel most important: to love, to peace, to teaching, to healing, to our spiritual growth and the spiritual growth of others.

Take a moment to think about why you are here and what you're dedicated to.

So, what do we still need to know before we take the step to open our crown chakra?

Free Meditation

On my computer I have a scan disk program I run every time I set up the computer to start work. Its function is to search for errors, clutter, bits of information stuck here and there. It cleans and tidies the disk, collecting like with like. It allows my computer to work faster and more cleanly, saving me time and frustration in the long run. Similarly, I have a machine in my swimming pool that goes around and eats leaves and debris that have fallen into the water to leave it clean and clear.

I see meditation as doing a combination of those things for my mind. It regularly sweeps up any mess I haven't cleared, relieving me of the burden of carrying it around and therefore unloading stress. And the amazing thing about it is I don't have to do anything except turn the program on and then relax. I don't have to think, organize, worry. I just close my eyes, focus for a moment on my breathing, enter into the meditational state and it all happens as if by magic.

But the best part is that not only is my mind clear and ready to work more efficiently on today's information and demands, but there are physical benefits accruing while I just sit there. My brain relaxes completely and even though it has the kind of brainwave pattern I'd have if I were asleep, I'm highly aware. My blood pressure comes down a little as does my heart rate, my breathing reduces in both rate and depth until I seem to be suspended in time and space and hardly needing any fueling at all. My mood automatically improves and any pain I may have had disappears. Afterward my reaction time is better, my memory is sharp, my thought processes are clear and I'm focused in an amazing way.

We've been doing guided meditations throughout our journey and I suggest that you continue to do these whenever you wish. It's good to continue to cleanse and balance your chakras in the way you've been doing, especially if for any reason you've felt upset or hurt. Please don't carry around any more baggage than you really have to. Remember our goal is to learn from all that happens, however painful it may be, and to turn it to our advantage—there always is one.

But now I'd like you also to experience the different kind of unrestricted meditation I've described above, if you haven't already done so. Millions of people have, ever since the Beatles put meditation on the map in the 1960s.

Getting into Alignment

We've been looking at the chakra system bit by bit to understand its functions, its gifts and perhaps why it hasn't been working as well as it might.

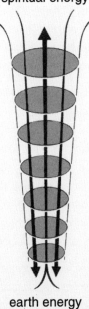

spiritual energy

earth energy

Figure 10

Now we can look at the system as a whole (see Figure 10). Here we have seven clear unobstructed chakras which form a series of hoops. We can see, and maybe feel, how easy it is to allow a breeze of energy to blow up and down through them all. We can experience the rise of energy from the earth and the incoming of spiritual energy from above. We can feel the amazing nourishment of that energy as it passes through but also shines out to fill us and to radiate beyond.

Holding onto that image, you can now attempt to transcend. Just close your eyes for a moment and visualize that core, as though there's an empty space through the middle of you, clear now as you've worked so hard on yourself. Allow yourself to feel pleased with yourself and let yourself rest now. Feel that free clear space and, with hardly any effort, allow it to fill with golden energy from the earth and white light from above. Allow yourself to smile inside as the energy just flows into the space you've made: feel it glowing and warm, like the gentlest of summer breezes, filling you now and making you whole in a totally new way. Just allow it to seep out into your tissues. Feel it healing everything. Feel it cleansing everything. Feel light and watch your mood begin to rise as you now have a kind of excitement in your solar plexus. Here it comes. Feel your spirituality. Feel it almost lift you off your seat. You're only held by your root chakra and you do need to hold on to that, but here you are now. You're about to transcend.

This is an experience that defies description. Just allow yourself to gently let go. You find yourself rising out through your crown chakra, out into clear space, beyond space. There's nothing, absolute nothingness. Just a mingling of you with your soul. Feel yourself rise now, and feel yourself gently lose all sense of your body as you gently blend now with that great body of spirit. Feel the ecstasy. Feel that sense of nothingness. Just be now. Just be. You hardly need to breathe. You need very little in material terms because your body is suspended and you are free in your spirit. You have transcended.

Stay for as long as you wish but when you're ready, you must return. This earthly plane is where you belong and you must come back and make a good connection again with your physical self. Come back through your crown chakra. Feel yourself inside your body. Begin to feel your weight on your seat. Feel your clothes on your skin. Feel your toes. Move them. Feel your fingers. Move them too. Now, be totally aware of your physical presence and, when you're fully back here, open your eyes.

Take a little time now before you continue. You may feel a bit spaced out and if you do, ground yourself again. Have a drink of water and perhaps a biscuit or a small snack so that your physical body has some work to do.

There's no need to try to record this experience unless you want to. It's often very difficult to put into words. If you didn't manage to let go and transcend, don't worry. Maybe you could try again using a pre-recorded audio-tape. Though silence is the best thing to help us transcend, some guidance is often necessary at first. You can do it, even though it might take some practice. I've never had anyone at a workshop who hasn't made it, though occasionally there's someone who isn't ready to try and that's absolutely fine. If you feel that way, you can always come back to this when you're ready.

If you did manage, you may now have a strange feeling around your heart chakra or in your solar plexus, or anywhere else for that matter. You might feel emotional and want to either laugh or cry. You may feel somewhat baffled and full of questions. You may feel in awe and wonder. Just take your time now before you do anything else. Plunging headlong into your day isn't a very good idea for ten minutes or so. Enjoy the feeling first and then be ready to begin again. You'll find that you're more alert, you feel loving, you want and are able to perform well.

Practice Channeling

Have another look at Figure 10. You can see that with all your chakras aligned and open, you have a tube, a channel, that's now clear and open. You can invite something to enter at the top and it will because now there's a clear space. But be aware. Prepare yourself well and don't rush ahead here.

When I want something to enter I especially ask before I begin that it will be the most pure, most loving, most healing, most high energy I can possibly have. I don't want just anything to flow through me.

Whether I'm doing this for myself or for someone else in a reading, or to help when I'm working with them, I want it to be as accurate as possible. I also want to get Brenda out of the way so that my thought processes don't interfere with what's coming through the channel I've cleared. That means I have to lovingly put Brenda aside, and what usually happens is that I can feel the essence of my earthly self stand a little to the left and slightly in front of me.

This sounds strange and it may be very different for you. But just focus for a moment on being divorced from what is about to happen so that you don't get your own life and thoughts involved with it. The more you can stand aside, the more accurate your reading will be.

Now, send up the message that you would like the highest possible wisdom, the purest possible healing, the most accurate information and then stand aside and wait. When you're adept at this, you'll find the stream opens up very quickly. But at first it may take time. You'll know when it's happening because you'll be almost an observer to it and be aware that it has nothing whatsoever to do with you.

The first time this happened to me, spontaneously and not using the method I'm describing, I was at a conference and got up onto the stage with my few notes, asked the divine as always that I'd give the audience what they most needed from me, and opened my mouth to begin. Suddenly I heard a very eloquent lecture being given that had nothing to do with me or with the notes I'd prepared. I never use my notes anyway, but I do have them there and I knew that what was coming out of my mouth was not only nothing I had prepared, it was far better than I could have done. I just stood there and listened and enjoyed the applause at the end while feeling like a bit of a fraud.

It was rather like I used to feel when I was little and healing just flowed. Now I've learned how to access that when I want it and not have it burst through if I don't. I can also now have it running simultaneously while I'm working so that I can have messages about what to do next or what the client needs to know now. I can "hear" the information and act on it while I'm still continuing to talk and listen to what the person is saying. Only sometimes does that become a little confusing and I have to stop for a moment and "listen" before I can proceed.

Many people who channel talk in terms of specific spirit guides. I mentioned some of the most publicized ones in Chapter 8. I don't perceive it in that way myself. Maybe I will some day, or maybe it's that I do a different kind of work and don't need it to be that way. I don't know. I'm just forever grateful that it happens as it does, and a steady flow of ready-formed information keeps pouring through me. My mouth speaks it while I just stand by. Sometimes I remember what's been said and sometimes I don't. It doesn't really matter.

If you're going to have a try at channeling, you'll need to have some recording device by you, whether a notebook and pen, a tape recorder or a friend you can trust to be there and scribe for you but without making any comment and certainly without bursting into laughter.

Please always begin by being grounded, by asking that you receive only the best and by trying to get yourself out of the way. That will come to you, I'm sure. Then allow yourself to be open, and let whatever happens happen. You may find that you have a stream of consciousness flow through you and then it seems to stop and you lose the connection. That's usually because your mind clicks in again and you get involved with what's going on. You'll be able to tell immediately if that happens. It's almost as though you hit the earth with a thud and you're back here feeling a bit foolish because you don't really know what you were talking about. That's okay. Just center yourself again, and off you go.

When you feel it's over for now, or you're tired and want to stop, all you have to do is think that and move back into place, and there you are. Give thanks. Get grounded again. Feel your physical body. Do all the usual things: have a drink of water and take your time before you do anything else.

A handy tip: while it's happening don't worry about what you're saying, what's going on, how accurate it might be or that you might be making a fool of yourself. If you do that, you'll immediately interfere with the process and lose the connection. However, until you've mastered the art, please don't attempt to channel anything for anyone else, because you may not be very accurate and may give them information that they believe. So please respect what's going on.

The other thing is to report it as it is. Sometimes there's an urge to attempt to make sense out of what's coming through. I've found that when that happens, the essence that was so important to the other person gets lost. Often when using angel cards (See Chapter 2), I get the "obedience" card and I'm sure that's to remind me to tell it as it is because that's how the client needs to hear it. It's none of my business to alter it, try to make it more palatable or doctor it in any way. I think your integrity will give you an uncomfortable time if you stray from what you know to be right.

ENLIGHTENMENT

This is a never-ending, ever-expanding, never to be completed, amazingly wonderful state that we can touch and explore, but that few of us will ever conquer in this lifetime. Nor perhaps in many lifetimes to come. Yet it's the state for which we are ever striving even before we're aware that we're doing so.

In saying all that, it may feel as though I got you here (or more accurately you got yourself here) under false pretenses. Here at the end of the rainbow there's no pot of gold after all. But there was gold all the way along the journey. You're more whole, more healthy, more real, more loved and loving. You're more open and have new (or rather have redeveloped old) skills and have left behind much that troubled you. You've offloaded old grief, pain and resentment, found a better way to live that has love at its heart, both human and celestial, and you know too much ever to go back to where you were.

But there's always more to know. More to explore, more to discover. And that's how it needs to be.

Final Meditation

The colors are white, purple and gold. Though you have all you need within yourself to complete this meditation, if you have something purple and regal, white and innocent or gold, set the scene by wearing it or take it to your safe place now.

The stones that are particularly useful here are diamonds, the master healers. This is the time to wear your diamonds, ladies. They purify the spirit and reflect the highest consciousness while inspiring innocence and serenity. Gold balances everything and helps aid illumination, so if you have a ring or other jewelry with a diamond set in gold, clean it and wear it.

Celestite, which I mentioned in the last chakra and which improves awareness of the divine, or white tourmaline which also helps connect to the highest consciousness, are also appropriate here, as is our old friend clear quartz. It aids meditation, communication and healing.

If you want to use your vaporizer or burn incense, amber is a good choice.

Go now to your safe place and take with you anything you wish. Though you may want to prepare yourself with music, the best thing for the crown chakra is silence. Although I feel it's important for you to do this final meditation here in your safe place, you may find that at another time you'd like to go somewhere inspiring where you can be in nature and away from your daily life. I like beaches, moors and woods. But be sure it's somewhere safe. Though by this point we're very protected, please be responsible and not foolhardy.

As usual, focus on your breathing, relax your body and let go of anything negative. Be focused within yourself. With great respect and reverence, take your focus up now to your crown chakra and with a single loving thought allow it to open, visualizing it as a beautiful crown of light above your head. Allow it to open and increase in circumference and feel the wonder and beauty of it. Allow yourself to send up love to the highest possible point and then welcome back down that beam of light and love, coming down and pouring in through your crown. Allow yourself to feel its radiance, feel its wonder.

Let it come down to your brow now, where it changes to a deep blue or violet. Feel yourself filled with wisdom, with understanding. Let it flow down to your throat where it changes to a beautiful sky blue or turquoise. Feel yourself filled with creativity, with truth, with integrity. Allow it to flow down to your heart now where it changes again to a wonderful green. Feel yourself filled and overflowing with unconditional love for yourself and for all the universe. Let it flow on down to your solar plexus where it becomes brilliant yellow. Feel yourself filled with power as your will is reinforced and you accept responsibility for the great being that you are. Let the light move on down to your sacral chakra where it becomes bright orange. Feel yourself as a powerful sexual being, capable of relating to others as an equal on any level. Finally, let the light fill your root chakra where it becomes ruby red as it fills your pelvis and holds you firm, rooting you to the earth from which your physical body came and to which it will eventually return.

Now, see yourself in all your radiance. See who you really are. Allow yourself a mixture of pride and humility at the wonderful creature you've become while still being a small part of a wondrous whole.

Breathe, breathe in the power and the majesty. Be who you are. Feel yourself fully alive. Just be.

Let the energies flow through you and around you. Let yourself be totally healed. Let no one ever take this from you. This is who you are. Enjoy. Just be.

Stay as long as you wish and, when you are ready, close down very carefully, protect all your chakras by putting around you that velvet cloak we mentioned in the protection exercise (see page 57), then once again begin to feel your physical presence. Start to gently move your toes and your fingers and, when you're ready, return to the room.

Have a drink of water and be sure that you're grounded before you get on with your day.

Final Message

So here we are at the end of our journey together. Or maybe not. There is still more journeying to do and, who knows, perhaps we shall do more of it side by side in the future. I have loved journeying with you.

I wish you love and joy, laughter and happiness, good companions with whom to travel, and a safe and wonderful journey home.

Appendix A: Endocrinological and Neurological Connections

༄

The interface between the chakras and the physical body occurs at the level of the major endocrine glands. The following is intended to be a simple and quick reference, not an endocrinological dissertation. If you want to follow up on any of this, I'd recommend that you either speak to your doctor or purchase a textbook.

If you have dysfunction in any of the areas mentioned, working on the appropriate chakra will help, though as always, please think very carefully before discontinuing or ignoring any medical advice you may have. Working with the chakras can be a beneficial adjunct to traditional treatment but is not meant to replace it.

Almost everything we do has a hormonal basis: having sex, going to sleep, becoming tearful, being angry, feeling our sexual identity, choosing our life partner, running away when we're scared or standing our ground to protect our young. And that's not to mention basically every physiological function from passing urine, maintaining your body temperature and regulating your salt and water balance to increasing your heart rate when you exercise. Without good control over our internal mechanisms, by the process known as homeostasis, our physical body gets into difficulties (dis-ease) and may die.

Endocrinological Connections

Root Chakra

Associated organ—Adrenal glands.

Functions—Two separate parts: the medulla and the cortex. The medulla secretes adrenaline, which acts directly on the heart, blood vessels, lungs and muscles in what is termed the fight-or-flight response. The cortex secretes steroids, which are essential for the balance of physical and emotional energy levels and for our response to shock and stress. It also produces aldosterone, which deals with water balance and the balance of sodium and potassium.

Malfunction—Under-functioning causes Addison's disease and hypoaldosteronism. Over-functioning causes Cushing's disease, hyperaldosteronism and excessive sex hormone production. The latter may cause difficulty in the development of the sexual organs or secondary sexual characteristics during puberty such as the development of breasts, body shape and the distribution of body hair, and also difficulties with menstruation and reproduction.

Sacral Chakra

Associated organs—Ovaries in women, testicles in men and the lymphatic system.

Functions—The ovaries and testes (the gonads) secrete hormones that are intimately involved with puberty, fertility, menstruation, pregnancy, menopause and sex drive (libido).

The lymphatic system is not an endocrine organ, but since it's so intimately involved with this chakra this seems a good place to mention it. Its functions include the transport of lymphatic fluid, of infective agents such as bacteria and of cells such as cancer cells. The glands, which are found throughout the body, swell up in infections as they provide a series of dams and locks to prevent the spread of disease. They form a major part of the physical body's defense system.

Malfunction—Problems with the gonadal system can cause difficulties with all the processes mentioned above, but also with the closure of the epiphysis (the growth plates of bones, which usually stop bone lengthening after puberty) and the development of osteoporosis.

Problems with the lymphatic system result in a breakdown of the body's defenses, recurrent infections, swollen glands and retention of fluid.

Solar Plexus Chakra

Associated organ—Pancreas.

Functions—The pancreas secretes two major hormones, insulin and glucagon, both of which are essential for carbohydrate metabolism. They have opposite effects and their balance is important in maintaining blood glucose levels. Glucose is the only food substance utilized by the brain and therefore the effect of insulin and glucagon on brain function is of major importance.

Malfunction—The major pathology associated with the pancreas is diabetes mellitus, though there may be more minor, but important fluctuations in blood sugar that can greatly affect our levels of physical energy.

Heart Chakra

Associated organ—Thymus.

Functions—These are still not fully understood, but the thymus is important in the development of the fetus and in the body's immune response, especially the production of T-cells.

Malfunction—This isn't completely understood either. Auto-immune diseases, the most commonly known now being AIDS, are affected by the thymus, as are some forms of cancer. In adults the thymus atrophies, usually beginning around the time of puberty, apparently in response to the increase in sex hormones secreted at that time. It appears to degenerate even more during each pregnancy and continues to do so throughout life.

Throat Chakra

Associated organs—Thyroid and parathyroids.

Functions—The thyroid gland affects metabolism in several ways— growth, temperature control, energy production and carbohydrate and fat metabolism. In babies it is also concerned with intellectual development.

The four parathyroid glands are essential to calcium metabolism, which is involved in bone and tooth health and also in the proper functioning of muscle, including heart muscle. It's also essential for the metabolism of Vitamin D, and has an action on the kidneys and also on the gastrointestinal tract.

Malfunction—The main features of hyperthyroidism (thyrotoxicosis) include rapid pulse, sweating, intolerance to heat, insomnia, excitability, nervousness, irritability, weight loss and irregular menstruation. The main features of hypothyroidism include depression, weight gain, coarsening of hair and skin, lethargy, hypersomnia (wanting to sleep excessively), intolerance to cold, and poor memory and concentration.

Hyper-parathyroidism's main features include headache and mental confusion, excessive thirst and urination, kidney and gallstones and calcification of the cornea.

Hypo-parathyroidism's main features include degenerative changes in bones, teeth and fingernails, and cataracts.

Brow and Crown Chakras

I've put these together because there's still some discussion as to which chakra is involved with which of these glands. They're so closely linked in the brain anatomically that I feel it is best to discuss them together. The wisdom I receive states that the pituitary and hypothalamus are associated with the brow and the pineal with the crown, but I greatly respect other sources who feel that it's the other way around.

Associated organs—Pituitary, hypothalamus and pineal glands.

Functions—The hypothalamus is a part of the brain that secretes hormones, which in turn regulate the flow of hormones from the pituitary. The pituitary gland regulates the whole endocrine system. It has two lobes, anterior and posterior. The anterior secretes a hormone that stimulates all the others in the endocrine system. The posterior stimulates the womb to contract in pregnancy and also initiates lactation (milk production).

The pineal secretes melatonin, which stimulates sleep and in animals governs migration patterns and hibernation. It appears to control our body clock and our daily biological rhythms. It may also have some effect on libido and maternal behavior and possibly on aging. It also has an effect on jet lag.

Malfunction—Since the pituitary orchestrates all the endocrine glands to some extent, its malfunction can affect pretty much every system of the body and its effects are too numerous to mention. Malfunction of the pineal may have an effect on sexual activity as well as causing sleeping difficulties.

Neurological Connections

As well as being intimately connected to a major endocrine organ, each chakra also has a connection with a nerve plexus, a ganglion or bundle of nerves coming together to supply a particular area, or in the case of the sixth and seventh chakras, the connection is with the brain itself. The sixth chakra also has a connection with the carotid plexus.

Root chakra—coccygeal plexus, which is a small plexus supplying the anal and genital region.

Sacral chakra—sacral plexus, which supplies the buttocks, thighs and lower limbs. It also has a branch to the anal sphincter.

Solar plexus chakra—gastric and hypogastric plexuses, which supply the digestive system.

Heart chakra—pulmonary and cardiac plexuses, which are to some extent an extension of each other and supply the respiratory tract, the heart, aorta and pulmonary vein.

Throat chakra—pharyngeal plexus, which supplies the throat area, the pharynx, the tongue and the palate. The brachial plexus, which supplies the arms, may also be involved.

Brow chakra—carotid plexus, which supplies fibers to the head, neck and ears.

Crown chakra—cerebral cortex, which of course commands everything.

Appendix B:
Evidence of Etheric Bodies

∿

For centuries, writings from a broad range of cultures and religions have referred to the presence of an energy field that extends from the physical body and is usually described as light.

There are ancient scrolls describing the aura as perceived by mystics and healers and there are dolls that have been found at ancient sites around the world that have the chakras clearly marked upon them.

Early Egyptian, Indian and South American literature and art all depict the presence of the aura and in some cases the chakras. The kaballah refers to the radiance as astral light, while early Christian writings and art witness the presence of haloes around the head, and in some cases the whole body, of religious figures. Within Hindu Vedic writings, theosophy, Buddhism and Native American teaching, there are also references to light emitting from the body.

From ancient Egypt there is support for this visual evidence in the fact that the kings wore special apparel to protect the chakras—note the false beard that protects the throat chakra and the high elaborate headgear with serpent at the forehead that protects the crown and the brow.

Yet, as we moved from ancient to modern times, people became more skeptical and less willing to accept the presence of auras and chakras without hard evidence.

Only in this century have we been well enough equipped to carry out properly designed and controlled studies to try to elucidate the mystery of the life force. In this pursuit, the energy field has been subjected to rigorous examination in terms of its consistency, its composition and its properties. Its electromagnetic and electrostatic properties have been measured, and its energy photographed by means of Kirlian photography. Dr. Valerie Hunt in the United States, who has specialized in this field for almost thirty years, has recorded electromagnetic radiations from the bodies of many subjects. There is now available video footage showing the aura and its changes in color and texture as the subjects photographed take part in different activities. The results are not only exciting, in that at last the aura can be quantified scientifically, but, more importantly, they at last validate the claims of the mystics and healers over the centuries whose integrity had been doubted and ridiculed. I would refer you to *Hands of Light* by Barbara Brennan, *The Chakras* by C. W. Leadbeater and *Wheels of Life* by Anodea Judith, in which you will find excellent accounts of research and evidence of the etheric bodies.

Glossary

Affirmations—positive statements in the present tense that allow us to visualize and eventually create a new reality. Affirmations help us shape our world and change our lives (see Chapter 8, page 173).

Astral plane—perhaps the most commonly known of the auric layers: that place we may experience in dreams, in near death experiences, in psychosis, in drug-induced experiences. It is a place some people float into when shocked or distressed, when they leave their bodies though still remaining attached and looking on as an observer. (In psychiatric terms this is known as depersonalization.) After death some souls remain for a while in the astral plane before releasing themselves to go to higher planes. In transcendence we pass through and rise above the astral and return through it again as we ground ourselves.

Autogenic training—a means of teaching yourself to change and a means of controlling those functions that most of us feel are involuntary, e.g. blood pressure, pulse rate.

Catharsis—a process whereby so-called negative emotions (sadness, anger, grief, etc.) which have been buried are brought to the surface and expressed.

Clairaudience—the psychic gift of hearing at vibrational levels usually beyond human perception. This is activated at the fifth (throat) chakra.

Clairvoyance—the psychic gift of seeing beyond what is commonly available to human perception. This ability is activated at the brow chakra.

DNA—deoxyribonucleic acid, a substance that exists as intertwining strands and holds coded genetic information which is unique and specific to any individual.

Ether—see Chapter 8, page 169

Hands-on healing—the method of healing where the healer actually touches the person (though without removing clothing). Sometimes also referred to as "the laying on of hands." Many healers hold their hands within the aura and don't make contact with the physical body.

To some extent this is a personal preference, though for me there are some instances where aura healing is more appropriate and at others I'm guided to touch.

Ida—one of the lateral energy channels (*nadis*) that twine around the central energy channel as represented in the caduceus (page 68). It represents the feminine.

Karma—cycle of cause and effect in which we eventually come to a state of balance. In simple terms, what we put into life we get out. What we sow, we reap. Karma is continuous through all our lifetimes.

Karmic connection—connection with a soul with whom we have reincarnated in the past and with whom we still have unfinished business. We may reincarnate with some of the same souls again and again until we have finished a mutual process of learning and teaching.

Karmic debt—this occurs where we have not come into balance at the end of one lifetime and we bring into the next some unfinished business that we still have to complete.

Kundalini—the energy stored in the root chakra, often symbolically represented as a snake, which when released opens and aligns the whole chakra system with a stimulation of powerful creative energy.

Mantra—words, phrases or sounds that we repeat internally or aloud as a tool to help change our consciousness and enter a meditative state (singular: mantram).

Pingala—one of the three central energy channels representing the masculine. Sometimes the two lateral channels, of which this is one, are referred to as the *nadis*.

Soul mate—a soul whom we have known over many lifetimes and with whom we have much in common in terms of characteristics and goals. Finding our soul mate doesn't mean we will always stay with them. The connection may be extremely deep and wonderful, allowing much to be completed for both partners so that they can move on. We can have more than one soul mate in a lifetime.

Sushumna—The central power channel that runs up through the region of the spine and connects the roots of each of the chakras. This is the channel through which the kundalini rises.

T-cell—specialized white blood cell, the T-lymphocyte, which is essential in the immune response. There are different categories, some of which help kill cancer cells, some of which stop the body from attacking its own cells and some of which process information.

Bibliography

Dr. Daniel Benor, *Healing Research—Holistic Energy Medicine and Spirituality*, Helix Editions, 1993.

Barbara Brennan, *Hands of Light*, Bantam Books, 1993.

Shakti Gawain, *Creative Visualization*, Bantam Books, 1983.

Gerald Jampolsky, *Love Is Letting Go of Fear*, Celestial Arts, 1988.

Anodea Judith, *Wheels of Life*, Llewellyn Publications, 1987.

Shafica Karagulla and Dora van Gelder Kunz, *The Chakras and the Human Energy Field*, Theosophical Publishing House, 1989.

Phyllis Krystal, *Cutting the Ties that Bind*, Samuel Weiser, Inc., 1994.

C. W. Leadbeater, *The Chakras*, Theosophical Publishing House.

Laurens van der Post, *A Story Like the Wind*, Harcourt Brace & Company, 1978.

Laurens van der Post, *A Far Off Place*, Harcourt Brace & Company, 1978.

Jane Roberts, *The Seth Material*, Buccaneer Books, 1995.

Sanaya Roman, *Living with Joy*, H. J. Kramer, 1986.

Ruth White, *Gildas Communicates*, Beekman Publishers.

Index

Other Ulysses Press Mind/Body Books

THE 7 HEALING CHAKRAS WORKBOOK: EXERCISES AND
MEDITATIONS FOR UNLOCKING YOUR BODY'S ENERGY CENTERS
Brenda Davies, M.D. $16.95
Filled with step-by-step guided activities—including meditations, ques-
tionnaires, creativity exercises and journal writing—this companion
workbook to *The 7 Healing Chakras* allows you to achieve your full
potential and improve virtually every aspect of your life.

CHAKRA POWER BEADS: TAPPING THE POWER OF ENERGY STONES
TO UNLOCK YOUR INNER POTENTIAL
Dr. Brenda Davies, $9.95
Explains how to improve health, spirit and fortune by fully harnessing
the power of beads.

UNLOCKING THE HEART CHAKRA:
HEAL YOUR RELATIONSHIPS WITH LOVE
Dr. Brenda Davies, $14.95
Applying the principles of the chakra system, *Unlocking the Heart Chakra*
examines the central relationships in our lives and offers a plan for
understanding them.

HEALING REIKI: REUNITE MIND, BODY AND SPIRIT
WITH HEALING ENERGY
Eleanor McKenzie, $17.95
Examines the meaning, attitudes and history of Reiki while providing
practical tips for receiving and giving this universal life energy.

HOW MEDITATION HEALS: A SCIENTIFIC EXPLANATION
Eric Harrison, $12.95
Combines Eastern wisdom with medical and scientific evidence to
explain how and why meditation improves the functioning of all
systems of the body.

HOW TO MEDITATE: AN ILLUSTRATED GUIDE TO CALMING THE
MIND AND RELAXING THE BODY
Paul Roland, $16.95
Offers a friendly, illustrated approach to calming the mind and raising
consciousness through various techniques, including basic meditation,
visualization, body scanning for tension, affirmations and mantras.

101 SIMPLE WAYS TO MAKE YOUR HOME & FAMILY SAFE IN A TOXIC WORLD
Beth Ann Petro Roybal, $11.95
Sheds light on common toxins found around the house and offers parents straightforward ways to protect themselves and their children.

SENSES WIDE OPEN: THE ART & PRACTICE OF LIVING IN YOUR BODY
Johanna Putnoi, $14.95
Through simple, accessible exercises, this book shows how to be at ease with yourself and experience genuine pleasure in your physical connection to others and the world.

SIMPLY RELAX: AN ILLUSTRATED GUIDE TO SLOWING DOWN AND ENJOYING LIFE
Dr. Sarah Brewer, $15.95
In a beautifully illustrated format, this book clearly presents physical and mental disciplines that show readers how to relax.

TEACH YOURSELF TO MEDITATE IN 10 SIMPLE LESSONS: DISCOVER RELAXATION AND CLARITY OF MIND IN JUST MINUTES A DAY
Eric Harrison, $12.95
Guides the reader through ten easy-to-follow core meditations. Also included are practical and enjoyable "spot meditations" that require only a few minutes a day and can be incorporated into the busiest of schedules.

YOGA IN FOCUS: POSTURES, SEQUENCES AND MEDITATIONS
Jessie Chapman   Photographs by Dhyan, $14.95
A yoga book unlike any other, *Yoga in Focus* could just as easily be a gift book as a tutorial. The presentation captures the very essence of yoga, combining perfectly positioned figures in meditative black-and-white photos.

To order these books call 800-377-2542 or 510-601-8301, fax 510-601-8307, e-mail ulysses@ulyssespress.com, or write to Ulysses Press, P.O. Box 3440, Berkeley, CA 94703. All retail orders are shipped free of charge. California residents must include sales tax. Allow two to three weeks for delivery.

About the Author

Dr. Brenda Davies, a British psychiatrist and spiritual healer, combines her traditional medical training with ancient healing gifts. Having lived and worked around the world, she now resides in Texas, though her workshops, clients and conferences keep her on an international circuit. A mother of two and grandmother of one, she is happily living her own spiritual path while exploring the frontiers of love and healing. She is currently writing her third book.